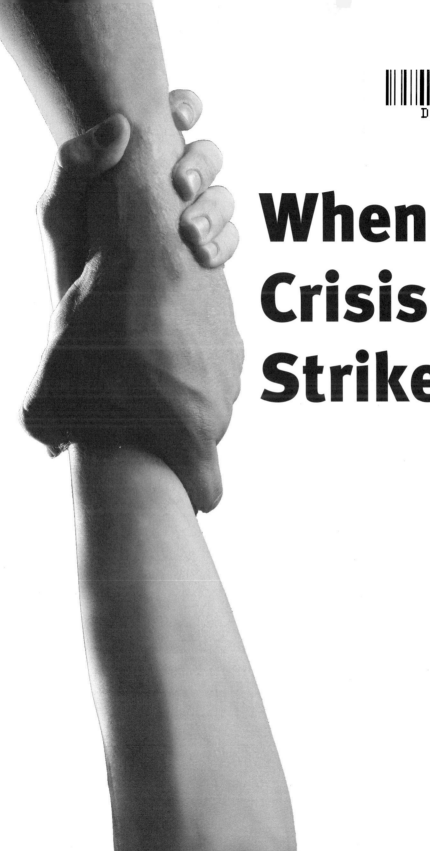

D1441009

When
Crisis
Strikes...

When Crisis Strikes...

What To Do
What To Say
How To Help

by
Allidah Poole Hicks
and
Bonnie Knuti

Good Neighbors Publishing LLC

When Crisis Strikes…What To Do, What To Say, How To Help

Editor: Barbara Munson, Munson Communications

Cover and Graphic Designer: Rebecca Finkel, F + P Graphic Design

Interior Layout Designer: Ronnie Moore, WESType Publishing Services, Inc.

Indexer: Madge Walls, All Sky Indexing

Published by:
Good Neighbors Publishing LLC

24325 Winder Place
Golden, CO 80403

www.WhenCrisisStrikes.com

ISBN 978-0-9824028-0-1

Library of Congress Control Number 2010907550

Caregiving, Health, Grief, Reference

Printed in the United States of America

10 9 8 7 6 5 4 3 2 1
First Edition

Acknowledgments

From Allidah...

I am truly a lucky person. I've always been surrounded by one loving community or another. From childhood, I've had the opportunity to see people put their love of God into action, to support and comfort those in their midst. And, I've always known that I could count on them should I need them. For these amazing gifts, I thank The Village Church of Western Springs, the Wheat Ridge Presbyterian Church, and the Shepherd of the Hills Presbyterian Church families.

And then, there are the Church Chix. Though now scattered about, we are threaded together by shared moments, limitless laughter, and Christian love. I've learned so much from these great women.

Every day I feel so fortunate to come home to the Field Drive neighborhood. The folks who live here are so giving and kind. It's these people who picked up Bonnie's (my co-author) family when her son Peter became ill. Off and on for years, they brought meals, tended the yard, took care of the pets, made home repairs, gave blood, and simply cared. What a wonderful, warm, and caring group of people! They're really something special.

My family has been my greatest life adventure. I am so grateful to my very talented and mellow husband David who has always encouraged me in this venture. Countless times over the last decade, he has "saved the day" when Bonnie and I have had computer disasters and he has dropped everything to weigh in on our endless editing and content debates. "Thank you" will never be sufficient for all his time and support. And, every day I thank God for our children, Brennan and Benay, who have brought us incredible joy as we've watched them grow into kind and caring people.

Then, there is my mom. An RN with a God-given mission, she has been my ultimate role model. Without fanfare, she has spent her life caring for those who are shut-in, lonely, and forgotten. I want to grow up to be like my mom.

Most importantly, this book is written as a tribute to some very dear people...to Janice Bostrom, a vibrant young girl, whose death so long ago changed me...to Kirsten Marine, whose life was stolen by a careless driver, leaving behind her husband Eric and her son Nick...to Sarah Clarkson and her family...to Holly Butler and her family...and to Peter Knuti, a spirited teen, who left us and his family, Bonnie, Lee, and Kristi, far too soon. Their personal stories and their courageous struggles to survive the hand they were dealt are the inspirations for this book.

From Bonnie...

Every inch of the way, my family has supported me through thick and thin. Words just can't say how much I love and appreciate them. A loving thanks to my husband Lee and to my daughter Kristi. A warm thanks to my parents, Anne and Chris, who have recently departed, and to my other dear family members, Anne and Emily, Molly and Eric, Dave and Joan, Chris and Kathy, Ann Knuti, and Anne Collins.

Thank you to Dr. Linda Stork whose brilliant medical expertise combined with her compassionate care carried all of us through such tough years of struggle.

Thanks to Beth Woodard for her kind and professional coaching. Thanks to Allidah Hicks and to Connie Hirz who continue to bring love and make a difference in people's lives.

From both of us...

Our book has certainly been a long road. We are grateful to the many who have helped us along the way. Dr. Judith Briles, armed with talent and publishing savvy, skillfully and patiently steered us throughout this publishing journey. Barbara Munson, our editor, provided kind input and advice. Rebecca Finkel was a delight to work with and designed our book with enthusiasm and a creative eye. Ronnie Moore magically and carefully formatted our manuscript into a book. And, Madge Walls artfully indexed our book to make it more user-friendly.

We are so grateful to Brian Luke Seaward, Ph. D., renowned author and teacher on health and wellness, who took his time to review our book in its infancy. His generous encouragement and wonderful suggestions all along the way have kept us going.

David Hicks and Lee Knuti, our husbands, stoically endured our constant ramblings and years of neglect. Nevertheless, they cheerfully provided key input along the way. There are no words that can truly express our gratitude.

A number of folks took time out to look over our book and give us valuable feedback. Thanks to Angie Augur, Mona Baxley, Emily Hassler, Allison Herron, Kristi Knuti, Laura Lang, Eric Marine, Sherri Michaelis, Ann Mullen, Anne Munch, Velma Poole, Warren Poole, Tilli Urban, Marilee Wehde, Molly Wittenberg, and Judy York. We are so grateful for their gifts of time and effort.

Along the way, we have both met all kinds of folks whose stories or pearls of wisdom have somehow been weaved into this book. To anyone we have missed acknowledging, you know who you are, and we thank you.

To my mother, Velma Just Poole,
who has always known
"the right thing" to do.

—Allidah Poole Hicks

To Lee and Kristi,
who live life with compassion,
and to Peter,
who showed us all how to "shine."

—Bonnie Knuti

Contents at a Glance

Table of Contents

Introduction

When it happens...

Everyone eventually gets that haunting phone call. In a flash, someone you know has been hit with a crisis...injured in an accident, faced with a tough diagnosis, limited by a debilitating condition, or crushed by the death of a loved one.

Our fears...

We all want to help in some way...say the right thing or do something that will make a difference. But, sometimes we get stuck, not knowing what to do.

❖ **We all worry that we might make a mistake.** So, we do nothing.

❖ **We're afraid we'll say something wrong.** So, we say nothing for fear our well-meaning words might sting.

❖ **Or, we don't step in to help at all because we know we can't fix it.** We think we have to do something big to really help.

❖ **Perhaps, we don't call or stop by for fear we might cry or fall apart.** We're afraid our tears might add to someone's burden.

❖ **And, worst of all, we might even find ourselves walking the other way.** It all feels "too close to home" and we worry that, somehow, we might catch this terrible plague of trouble.

Some truths...

But, here is what we have learned to be true.

❖ **Doing nothing is the biggest mistake we can make.** So, try something.

❖ **A heartfelt "I'm sorry" can usually clear the air if we accidentally hurt someone.** So, say something.

❖ **The smallest things can make a real difference.** A smile, a touch on the arm, a nod across a room, and a listening ear can mean the world to someone who's feeling alone.

❖ **Shedding a tear is human.** It shows that we have some understanding of how deeply our friend must hurt.

❖ **Trouble isn't contagious.** Bad things just happen to most of us at one time or another.

So...

If you have picked up this book, you have probably already gotten that haunting phone call. And now, you are struggling, just like we have, with that nagging question, "What can I do to help?" This book is full of ideas to get you started or to add to your collection of favorites. We applaud you for being there for your friends and family. You truly will make a difference.

Why we wrote this book...

Allidah's story

Much of my story cannot be told. Like so many, I protect a family member who suffers from a "sensitive illness." Our family knows what it is like to struggle alone with a disease that is neither well understood nor fully treatable. The aloneness my husband and I felt when the disease was raging and our loved one was hospitalized was unbearable. But, in the midst of this sorrow, our friend, Tom Wier, came to the door with a pizza, a listening ear, and a smile, and that moment made all the difference.

Several years later, an almost endless streak of tragedies hit people very close to our family. Peter, Bonnie's son, was diagnosed with cancer at age eleven and then struggled to survive for five years.

A woman speeding down the highway slammed her car into two others. In an instant, she destroyed two families. In one car were our closest friends. Kirsten was killed instantly and her husband, Eric, and their son, Nick, were severely injured. The other family had a similar fate, leaving a widow to pick up the pieces.

Sarah, a 12 year old from the girls' club I volunteer with, was hit by a car after school and landed in the intensive care unit. And then, my 41-year-old friend, Holly, had a damaging heart attack and bypass surgery.

Each time the phone rang, bringing devastating news, I struggled to do and say the right things. Sometimes I knew I made a difference; sometimes my gestures were clumsy; other times, I just didn't do enough, or I found I did too much. But, in the end, I learned that it's most important to just be there.

It's my hope that the stories and ideas shared here will be a jumping off place. Life will inevitably come tumbling down, but as we look for ways to reach out to each other, the possibilities for making a difference can be as varied as those who peek between the covers of this book.

Bonnie's story

My life took a dramatic turn for the worse on September 29, 1993, when my son, Peter, was diagnosed with Ewing's Sarcoma, a rare and very aggressive form of bone cancer. To say that my peaceful world was turned upside down is a gross understatement. For the next year, my husband Lee, my daughter Kristi, and I struggled as Peter underwent chemotherapy and several surgeries. In an effort to save his leg, Peter continued to endure repeated surgeries over a four-year period. It is no small exaggeration to say that all of us went through five years of unbelievable agony.

Just when we thought we were turning a corner, in the fall of 1997, Peter was diagnosed with AML leukemia, most likely a result of the initial chemotherapy. Although he put up a gallant effort, he did not survive the bone marrow transplant needed to cure the leukemia. Peter died on April 8, 1998, at the age of 16.

Peter's death just wrenched my soul. I guess it cracked my guard, allowing love and compassion to pour in. Up until that first shocking diagnosis, I would help others out of concern or obligation, but I really didn't fully understand how much people could make a difference to shattered lives.

During this ordeal, the outpouring of love from family, neighbors, friends, and colleagues was wonderful and certainly helped us navigate the shoals of some very rough seas. Given how busy everyone's life is in this fast-paced world, I was surprised by so much help.

When a friend, an acquaintance, or even someone we've never met struggles through the hazy nightmare of a jolting crisis, or the exhausting reality of enduring with an illness, I think most of us want to do something to help. When we ease the struggle and pain just a bit by jumping in to do what needs to be done to "keep the home fires burning," or when we support with genuine, loving words, I believe that we truly do make a difference.

How to use this book...

When we first began this book, we hoped it would give lots of ideas to folks who want to help someone struggling with a health crisis or a death. However, you will find that some of these ideas can also apply in other unhappy situations, such as the trauma of a divorce, or the loss of a job, home, or pet.

Feel free to start at the beginning of the book or with any chapter that interests you. For example, if a crisis has just struck someone you know, you can start at the first chapter, "Supporting when the crisis strikes…," and follow along as the person recovers. On the other hand, if you simply want to write an encouraging note to someone, you can go directly to Chapter 10, "Writing the right note…," and find an easy step-by-step formula.

Be sure to look through the **Table of Contents**. Perhaps you'll discover additional suggestions for helping now and later.

Sprinkled throughout the chapters are ***Care Tips*** that highlight important points. There are also ***Stories*** that show how helpers have made a difference for someone going through a difficult time.

Notice that each chapter begins with an ***Imagine,*** a question you might have when wanting to help someone. Each chapter ends with three different answers to that question. The ***Now imagine*** is a simple solution that only requires one person and a little window of time. The ***Or imagine***

xxviii   When Crisis Strikes...

requires a bigger gift of time, and the ***Or imagine this*** solution involves more time and more people.

You'll find that the book is organized into five parts. Each one speaks to different concerns that supportive people may encounter.

Part I, Helping along the road of life..., gives a picture of what the helper might face throughout the patient's journey to recovery. You'll find ideas for how to help when the crisis first strikes, throughout a hospital stay, during the homecoming, and then throughout the recovery period. Part I ends with a chapter on how to comfort the grieving when someone has died.

Part II, Caring with true kindness..., deals with the importance of protecting a person's privacy and not forcing your personal opinions and judgments on someone who is already facing a tough situation. Part II also includes valuable tips on what to say and what not to say to folks who have been struck by a crisis.

Part III, Everyday gestures..., answers the question, "What can I do to help?" It provides complete instructions for bringing snacks or a meal to an individual or family. It also shows you how to choose a gift with a special purpose in mind. You will also find detailed instructions for how to write a sympathy or encouraging note.

Part IV, Bigger efforts..., shows how to pull people together to help for a big event. You'll learn how to plan for a blood drive, fundraiser, or a reception after a death. In addition, you will see detailed instructions for providing food on a larger scale, an important ingredient for any event.

Part V, Additional resources..., provides useful forms that can organize and simplify the effort when many folks are involved. Feel free to go to our website, *www.WhenCrisisStrikes.com*, to download printer-friendly copies of each form.

Unfortunately, health crises will always be a part of the human road. We would all like to wave a magic wand and make people better, but we can't. We can, however, walk along side, offering a bit of comfort to people's troubled lives. It is our hope that this book will arm you with the tools you will need to reach out and make a difference in the lives of people around you.

CHAPTER ONE

Supporting when the crisis strikes...

In this chapter you'll find answers to...

- How do you begin to help when a crisis strikes?

- Who needs to know what's happened?

- What information should be shared?

- What can you do when long distance is an issue?

Imagine...

The phone rings. Something terrible has happened to your dearest friend. You are asked to come to the hospital right away. You want to help, but you don't know what you will find when you get there, what you should take that will be helpful, or what you should do.

When the crisis hits—what to do first...

When the phone rings, delivering very bad news about a family member or a close friend, time seems to just stop. Suddenly, all of your deadlines and your hectic schedules may be forgotten. The initial shock can feel the same regardless of whether the news is about a severe injury (auto accident, work-related trauma, burn) or a severe sudden illness (heart attack, stroke, devastating diagnosis).

Where is the crisis occurring?

We commonly think of a crisis occurring only at a hospital. However, a crisis usually affects people in several different places all at the same time. For example, with a terrible accident, someone may be whisked away to the hospital emergency room, while the parents at home receive the dreaded knock at the door, and the loving grandmother in another state gets the news in a shocking phone call. All of these people have just been hit by the same crisis and need help.

Sizing up the situation...

If you are one of the first at the scene (hospital, home, far away with someone hearing the news), pause to assess what's going on. Take a look at the whole picture.

Ask yourself:

❖ **Who is already at the scene? Who needs to be there?** Sometimes it isn't the obvious. Sometimes, family members want a special person (close personal friend, minister, spiritual leader) with them.

❖ **Is anyone in charge?** Maybe family members at the scene are totally overwhelmed. They may not know what they need or where to start.

Is anyone there thinking about what needs to be done or are they all too upset?

❖ **What has to be taken care of right way?** Do kids need to be picked up at the day care before it closes for the day? Does the dog need to be let out or fed? Does someone need to be notified immediately (work, school, team)? Do travel arrangements need to be made?

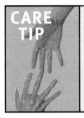

CARE TIP	No matter what you find at the scene, it's important to remain calm and collected. If you're too upset, find someone else who will stay levelheaded. The family does not need to take care of *you* during this difficult time.

What needs to be done right away?

A crisis takes everyone by surprise. Family members can be anywhere and everywhere. A mother could be at the office, a dad out of town, the children playing at a sport event, and the family pet cooped up in the home. A crisis offers a chance to make a difference — to jump in and help right away. Ask yourself, "What does this family need first? Do they have someone who is there and taking charge?"

If someone has "taken charge," then offer to assist.

❖ **Assist the family spokesperson who is an obvious leader.** This person may have already begun to call family and friends, ordered in food for hungry family members, made travel arrangements, and found someone to get essential items from the home. Offer to help in any way possible.

Ron's story

Ron, your very close friend, has been severely injured in a construction accident when a beam fell and knocked him out. He is now in a lengthy surgery.

You arrive at the hospital to find the family in the surgical waiting room, supporting Ron's wife, Cindy. Cindy's brother, Doug, is obviously in charge. He has already notified all of the family members and ordered take-out pizza for them all.

Though the needs of everyone at the hospital seem to be taken care of, you know that Ron and Cindy have a dog, a cat, and two birds at home. You offer to take care of the pets and anything else that might need attention at home, leaving them to focus on Ron and the family's needs at the hospital.

If no one has "taken charge," become the leader.

❖ **Calm the anxious.** When bad things happen, of course people are going to be upset. Sometimes, they will just need the right person to sit and listen to them and give them timely updates of the situation. Or, they might want your help to send a family member or friend, who may be kind but draining, on an errand.

❖ **Sort through the chaos.** Often family and friends will congregate and be so distressed that they don't know what to do next. In this case, offer to organize help. ***Always get permission from a key family member first.***

EXAMPLE: "School is getting out soon. Someone needs to pick up Susie. Would you be comfortable with me going to the school to get her, or do you have another plan?"

EXAMPLE: "It's getting close to dinnertime and you have all been here a long time. I would like to… (order some take-out food, get someone to bring over a dinner, bring in some sandwiches and fixings) for all of you so you don't have to think about it." (See "Navigating the hospital maze" on page 35 for other ways to help.)

❖ **Gather vital family members or friends.** Don't make assumptions that all of the "right folks" are there. In times of stress, people may not necessarily look for support from a family member, but maybe from someone who is a calming influence, a spiritual leader, or a friend who has experienced a similar crisis. *Ask.*

◆ **Let in-town family know.** Close family members should be notified *carefully*. Perhaps a child is at school, a wife is at work, or a parent is coming home from work and will be unaware of what has happened. Get input from the family to determine who will inform family members and what will be said. Be sure a trusted family member, a close friend, or a religious leader delivers the news personally in case anyone becomes distraught.

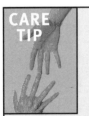

CARE TIP

Should you just assist the family or "take charge"? There is a fine line between helping and intruding. What's helpful for one family may be seen as intrusive to another. Also, what is helpful now might not be helpful down the road. It's not a matter of what's right or wrong. It's a matter of what fits for the family at the time. If you are unsure, remember to ask first.

1

- ◆ **Let out-of-town family know.** In some situations, an immediate family member may either live out of town or be out of town temporarily (school, business, vacation). Likely, he or she will become upset at the news and may need help making arrangements to get back home. If this is the case, try to find someone compassionate (school official, chaplain, nurse, counselor, hotel manager, police, fireman) who can either deliver the news or be with them as they receive it by phone.

- ◆ **Offer to drive or escort them if necessary.** It is best that distraught family members not drive immediately after receiving shocking news. They may not be able to drive safely or to find an unfamiliar hospital, especially if it's dark out. Out-of-town close family members may need someone to help make travel arrangements and even escort them.

❖ **Ask if there is anything the person or family wants done immediately.** What's first on *their* list is most important. Maybe they have concerns or responsibilities you wouldn't have even thought about or known about (carpool arrangements, commitments at work, pet care).

❖ **Determine if the children need care.** Find out where the children are. Do they need to be picked up or taken somewhere? Is someone carpooling them home? Will someone be home waiting for them if you cannot contact the driver? If young children are at the hospital, do they need to be entertained or taken to a waiting room? For some families, children can be a comfort in the midst of a crisis; for others, they are not. Children often are forgotten when a crisis is under way.

Clem's story

Clem, a friend from Rotary Club, had a stroke this afternoon. You head over to the hospital to check on him and to see if there's anything you can do. You meet his aging mother, Judy, who came by taxi as soon as she heard.

Clem will be in intensive care for quite some time and can only have close family visitors. Since Judy won't leave the ICU area, you go down to the cafeteria to get her something to eat.

Before you go, you ask Judy if there is anything else she needs done right away. She says she would love to have her good friend, Sarah, wait with her, but Sarah doesn't drive. You offer to pick her up.

Judy also remembers that she forgot to bring along her blood pressure medication that she takes twice a day. When you pick up Sarah, you'll also stop by Judy's house to get her medication.

Be sure to:

◆ **Entertain the children.** Little ones might get fidgety out of boredom or from the tension they absorb from the adults. Consider just playing quiet games with them, telling them stories, or just holding them. *Never take the children out of the parents' sight without a parent's permission.*

◆ **Provide any necessary transportation.** If the children have lessons, practices, or activities that the parents want continued during this stressful time, offer to get them there. *Again, no one should take the children without a parent's permission.*

◆ **Find safe childcare.** Small children are not usually allowed in emergency, surgical, or intensive care areas. Also, family members may not be able to focus on caring for children at this time. If this is the case, call a person *of the family's choosing* to care for them.

◆ **Explain the circumstances to the children.** If the immediate family members can't talk to the children at this time, perhaps they would like another relative or other trusted adult to tell the kids what has happened. Again, *always get a parent's permission as well as his or her input about what should be said.*

Anne's story

Your coworker, Anne, was so excited about the upcoming birth of her third child. When the baby started having trouble during labor, Anne had an emergency C-section and delivered a baby girl with many birth defects. She and her husband, Jim, had planned to bring the other children to see the new baby and for him to take care of them while Anne was in the hospital.

Given the circumstances, Jim wants to stay with Anne now. You offer to take care of the other two children until Anne comes home from the hospital.

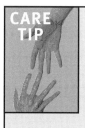

CARE TIP Encourage children to use other outlets (draw pictures, write letters, create cards, play catch, go for a walk, go out to eat and talk, tell stories about the injured or sick person, pray) to deal with their fears and their grief. *Only do this with a parent's permission.*

❖ **Ask if family members and friends at the scene need food or beverages.**
Because they are numbed by the crisis, they may not realize how long
it has been since they have had anything to eat or drink. Family and
close friends need to be encouraged to eat well and to drink plenty
of fluids during a time of crisis to keep up their strength.

◆ **In a hospital,** water, juice, tea, coffee, or hot chocolate is sometimes
free and available in the waiting rooms. If not, pick up something
on your way to the hospital or buy drinks from the cafeteria or
vending machines. Ideally, you have brought snack items with you.
(See "Feeding the body and soul" on page 165 for more ideas.)

◆ **At home,** just routinely offer beverages and healthy snacks. If the
pantry is empty, ask someone to make a quick run to the store,
or arrange for food delivery.

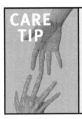
CARE TIP Divide up the work. Determine which person is best suited for each job (care for kids, run errands, stay with the patient or family members, get items from the family home). *Always get suggestions from the family.*

❖ **Ask if family members need a break.** Check to see how long they
have been there.

◆ **In the hospital,** offer to stay with the sick person or stay in the
waiting room awaiting news while family members leave for a
bit. Sometimes just a short break (bathroom, cafeteria, walk
around the block) makes all the difference.

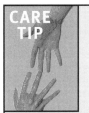

CARE TIP

In surgical or critical care waiting rooms, family members may be hesitant to leave for fear they will miss an important update about their loved one. Sometimes, they are so upset, they feel they cannot eat. Offer to stay while they take a break, assuring them that you will locate them immediately if anything happens or if a health-care professional wants to speak to them. Or, consider bringing in small portions of easy-to-eat snacks if they have no appetite at the moment.

1

◆ **At home,** family members will still need breaks. Offer to take over for a while (answer phones, greet visitors at the door, tend to the sick family member) while the caregiver takes a break (takes a nap, has a bit of privacy, handles business affairs, makes phone calls).

❖ **Does the patient or family need items from home?** In an emergency, people are not going to have their important items with them (medication, contacts case, eye glasses, toothbrush, comb). Offer to pick up these supplies from the patient's or family's home. (See "Personal Items Checklist For Helpers Staying Overnight" on page 41.) Since someone may have to go through personal drawers or cabinets, be sure the family trusts the person going into the home.

❖ **Is anyone caring for the family pets?** During a crisis, pets are often forgotten. But, remember, for many people, pets are their only companions and are beloved members of the family. Be sure someone is in charge of caring for them. Some pets will need frequent and immediate care; others can go unattended for a day or two.

Who else needs to know?

Letting in-town people know...

In the midst of a crisis, it's easy to forget that others who work or frequently play with the individual or family may need to know what's happened. Remember to contact them.

❖   Employers (including the teenager's job)

❖   Neighbors

❖   Insurance company

❖   Child-care facility

❖   School

❖   Church

❖   Sports teams

❖   Business clients

❖   Business associates

See form "Letting People Know" on page 303.

Letting out-of-town people know...

Sometimes, it's the folks who live far away who can provide the most support for the patient or family. With our mobile world, most of us still stay in touch with others who live in distant places. Don't forget to tell them because they will want to know and can sometimes be a huge support even from far away.

❖   Relatives

❖   Friends

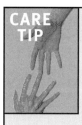

CARE TIP Find someone who is willing to loan a pre-paid phone card, a cell phone with unlimited minutes, or a computer for Internet calls. Perhaps someone is linked to a company or organization that can arrange for the family to use a free long distance telephone line temporarily.

1

❖ Business associates

❖ Business clients

❖ Old neighbors

❖ Previous church family members

❖ Previous schools

What should be told?

If the family has asked you to spread the word, you will need to gather some important information. Get *the key facts,* not all of the nonessential details. Be sure to write everything down so you can give the same information to everyone.

Getting the key facts...

❖ **What happened?** People you have been asked to notify and those who wish to help will want to know what has happened. Prepare to give a *simple and clear* explanation.

❖ *General condition* **of patient if known** (conscious, unconscious, in surgery) Remember, immediate details may not be available and they are not necessary to get help started.

❖ **Name of hospital** Due to the nature or severity of the injury or if the emergency room is crowded, the sick or injured may be taken to a different hospital than anticipated.

❖ **Location of hospital** Often hospitals have numerous sites. Get the address of the specific location.

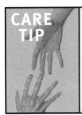 Even if details about the crisis are still sketchy, it's still possible to get the ball rolling and to get help on its way. You may be asked lots of questions, but unless specifically directed by the family, ***don't share details.***

❖ **Phone number in hospital where calls may be received** Ask the staff at the hospital where incoming calls can be received. Cell phones are often not allowed in a hospital due to sensitive equipment. Check first.

Sharing only the basics...

❖ **Keep explanations simple.** For example,

♦ "There was a car accident. John has many serious injuries and is in surgery. We'll know more later."

♦ "He had a stroke and now is paralyzed on the left side. He's in the Intensive Care Unit."

♦ "The baby was born with many birth defects and is having trouble breathing. They moved her to the Intensive Care Nursery."

Matt's story

Matt, a 35-year-old plumber and father of three young children, was on a job when he suffered a severe heart attack. He was not found right away, and was unconscious but still breathing when he was rushed by ambulance to the main city hospital.

His wife, Joan, calls you and is obviously very distraught. When you arrive at the hospital to support her, you ease her burden by agreeing to tell family and close friends about Matt's condition.

So that you don't forget to tell folks the essential information, you make a list of who needs to be notified and the basic important facts you want to tell them. Before calling anyone, you show Joan what you've written so she can check it over and make changes.

She also asks that Betty, a neighbor and close friend, pick up the three kids from school and day care. However, Joan wants be the one who tells her children the seriousness of their dad's condition. She asks that Betty only tell the kids that their dad got sick at work and had to go to the hospital.

◆ "She has died of a massive heart attack. We will notify you about services or receptions and let you know how you can help once the family has had time to make decisions."

❖ **What do you do when people press you for more information?** Inevitably someone will ask for more information than you should share. Plan ahead how to handle this situation. Consider saying, "That's all we know for right now. The family will tell us all more later."

Amanda's story

Amanda, a sixteen year old, committed suicide. Sandy, her mother, is heartbroken. As her closest coworker, Sandy wants your help telling the sad news and asks you to make all the necessary calls. You begin by finding out from Sandy who needs to be notified, both in-town and out-of-town.

The hardest part for Sandy is deciding what she wants people to know. As you talk together, Sandy finally decides to tell the least amount of information to the folks in town, as she really has no close ties with any of them.

When you call Sandy's work to tell them that Sandy's daughter has died, the boss is shocked, wants to help, and also wants to know more details. You say, "That's all I know for now. I will get back to you when I know more about a service and burial arrangements."

❖ **Welcome all offers to help.** When you notify people about the situation, many will ask how they can help. Be ready with suggestions and sign them up immediately! Perhaps they can help get kids to activities, house out-of-town family members who are coming to the hospital, or fire up their ovens and start baking.

How to help when the crisis is happening out of town...

Every crisis has ripple effects. With every local crisis, there will likely be some people living far away who will need support. It might be a parent

1

who needs to get to the bedside of his or her college student who has been in an accident. Perhaps a dear friend is asked to travel to another state to give the eulogy at a memorial service. Maybe a grandmother is needed to care for her grandchildren so the parents can be free to attend to a very sick child in the hospital.

When most people get the dreaded phone call that something bad has happened, they stop everything. Their only worry is to get to the scene where they are needed.

Find out if folks who live out of town need help making travel arrangements. Ask if they also need help with things at home (tending to animals, turning lights on and off, picking up newspapers, bringing in the mail) while they are gone. If folks are physically unable to leave, they will need support right where they are.

Getting folks to the scene...

Make emergency long distance travel arrangements. Investigate schedules and prices by phone or Internet. Find out about emergency rates. Assist the person in making final arrangements since they will likely be distracted.

❖ **Connect with someone at the scene who can help with out-of-town arrangements.** Is there a friend or neighbor at the scene who is willing to help answer questions or make arrangements for in-coming family and friends?

Find someone who will:

◆ **Arrange for pickup or transportation once they arrive at their destination.** Perhaps by talking with the family, friends, or neighbors at the scene, you can find someone to meet them at the airport, train, or bus station.

◆ **Suggest housing/motel arrangements.** Perhaps neighbors or friends, hearing of the problem, will offer their home or find someone else who can assist with a place to stay. Or, they will likely know about a nearby motel that will be clean, safe, and convenient.

❖ **Get them packed and ready to go.** With our busy lives, most of us wouldn't have our clothes ready to go. So, in an emergency, it might seem impossible to get packed and out the door. Help with the tasks that will make packing easy.

◆ **Wash clothes.** With permission, wash and dry the essentials, anything that needs to be packed.

◆ **Run to the dry cleaners.** If they request a special outfit that needs dry cleaning, look for 1-hour service.

◆ **Clean and polish shoes.** This small detail could be important in some families, especially if there's a chance that he or she will need to attend a funeral.

◆ **Borrow clothes appropriate for a memorial service.** Sometimes, people will say that they don't have an outfit or accessories (suit, dress, ties, dark shoes and socks) that are appropriate for a memorial service or funeral. You might call around to friends who are willing to loan an item or two. Don't forget to find clothes for the children who will be attending the service as well.

❖ **Help them get "out the door."** Call a taxi for them or drive them to the airport. Sometimes, a friendly face bringing reliable support can be such a warm comfort.

❖ **Escort them, if necessary.** Some people (elderly, frail, disabled) have a difficult time negotiating an airport, train station, or bus depot. They may need assistance getting a wheelchair, finding the right departure gate, getting to connecting flights, or using public restrooms. Offer to travel with them or arrange for an escort.

Taking care of things while they are gone...

❖ **Care for the animals.** This might mean running the pets to a kennel at the owner's request or you tending to them.

Mabel's story

Mabel, a 76-year-old woman, gets word that her adult son has been in a terrible car accident. She is devastated and does not know what to do first.

Sarah, her friend, knows that Mabel needs someone to stay with her, help her make emergency travel arrangements, and help pack. Sarah gets on the phone with the airline, explains the situation, and makes a reservation for the next morning. She also arranges for a wheelchair and special assistance to help her maneuver through the large airport. Sarah calls the son's best friend and he arranges to have someone meet Mabel at the airport. He also says that he'll be sure she's well taken care of while she's there.

With Mabel in tears, Sarah helps her sort out what she will need to take with her. She starts washing a load of laundry and makes a list of things Mabel will need to find and pack.

❖ **Make calls to inform people.** When someone has to leave right away, he or she probably won't have time to notify folks (work, family, friends, carpool drivers).

❖ **Assure them that their home will be cared for.** To prevent break-ins, make the house look lived in. Either do it yourself or find help to:

Either do it yourself or find help to:

◆ Water the indoor plants.

◆ Turn lights on in the evening.

◆ Shovel the snow-covered walks.

◆ Collect the mail and newspapers.

◆ Mow the grass.

◆ Rake the leaves.

Supporting those unable to leave...

❖ **Stay and keep them company.** Offer to stay at the home until another friend arrives to relieve you.

❖ **Call a religious leader or close friend.** Contact these people and get support going.

❖ **Offer something to eat and drink.** If the person is very upset, be sure to pay attention to the basics. Provide a simple meal.

1

❖   **Ask about medications.** Sad and upset people may forget to take routine medications. Remind them.

❖   **Contact people at the scene for the latest updates.** It may take someone levelheaded to stay in contact and gather information.

Note to helpers...

To be sure all of your support is truly kind,
take a look at Chapter 6, "Caring without offending"
and Chapter 7, "What *to* say, what *not* to say."

Now imagine...

Sirens blare as rescue workers enter your older neighbor's apartment.

Mrs. Alvarez has had a severe heart attack, is unconscious, and is being taken to the nearest hospital.

Although you don't know her well, you have chatted with Mrs. Alvarez frequently when you have seen her in the hall. Other than that, you are pretty sure she has been alone and has no close relatives or friends.

You know that the apartment manager will close the apartment and take care of the mail. However, he says that he doesn't know what to do about her pet bird. You offer to take the bird to your place until she returns.

When you call the hospital for an update of her condition, you hear that Mrs. Alvarez is being transferred from the Cardiac Care Unit to a semi-private room. You decide to visit her to let her know that you are caring for her bird, Pete.

Mrs. Alvarez seems so grateful for your visit and that you are looking after Pete. When you return, the nurse comments about how often Mrs. Alvarez has mentioned your kind visit. You really hadn't realized how meaningful such a small gesture could be.

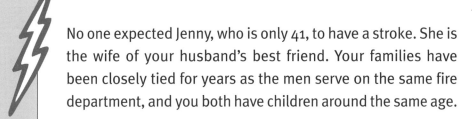

Or imagine...

No one expected Jenny, who is only 41, to have a stroke. She is the wife of your husband's best friend. Your families have been closely tied for years as the men serve on the same fire department, and you both have children around the same age.

When you arrive at the hospital, John, one of the off-duty firemen, is already organizing help at the hospital. Since your families are so close, he's counting on you to pick up the kids and to keep them until the grandmother arrives from out of town.

Or imagine this...

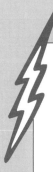

Your friend Carol's son, Mack, broke his neck playing football this afternoon. He's taken by ambulance to the hospital and you and Carol follow behind in your car. Mack is in the ER, will undergo some important tests, and will be taken to surgery. They fear he may be permanently paralyzed.

Carol is single and her parents live out of state. As her closest friend, you know that you need to jump in to organize help. You know the football booster club folks will be anxious to do whatever they can. You even figure that the football players can help, too.

First off, you need to find someone to take care of Jared, Mack's little brother. You're hoping that he can stay at his friend's house for a few days. You call to arrange care for Jared.

You ask the coach to coordinate a few players on the team to pick up the newspapers each morning, pick up the mail, and shovel the walk.

Since Carol will be staying with Mack continuously, you ask the president of the booster club to find someone to organize meals to be brought in to the hospital.

You need to go into work Monday through Friday, so you make sure someone is staying with Carol to support her. You stop in after work each day for as long as you can and make sure the help keeps on coming.

Navigating the hospital maze...

2

In this chapter you'll find answers to...

- What could you see at the hospital?

- How do you find your way around the hospital?

- What can you do to help at the hospital?

- How can you be a good visitor?

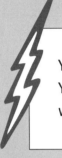

Imagine...

Your neighbor will be entering the hospital for a major surgery. You would like to be of help in some way, but you are not sure what you should do.

What to expect at the hospital...

If the crisis involves hospitalization, you'll need to consider some factors before you can be helpful. Every situation is different. You may find that the patient is alone in the room, or that one or more family members have arrived, or that numerous family and friends have gathered in a waiting room.

When a crisis hits, people often respond unpredictably. Someone who was once organized and dependable might now be too numb to make even the simplest decisions. Someone who was once levelheaded might now fly off the handle at the slightest irritation or be found laughing one minute and crying the next. Expect the unexpected!

The patient may...

❖   **...have had major surgery or some medical procedures.** The patient may look just fine or she or he may be attached to numerous tubes and equipment.

❖   **...be frightened, confused, or in pain.** On the other hand, the patient may still look and sound normal, but be in a great deal of distress.

❖   **...not act like himself or herself.** Sometimes injuries, illness, pain, treatments, or medication can affect a person's behavior. He or she may say odd, angry, or funny things and not remember them even a minute or an hour later.

Aunt Helen's story

Your refined Aunt Helen slipped and fell in her home, breaking her hip. The doctor has scheduled her surgery for tomorrow morning. You go to her hospital room and find her in a hospital gown, crying. Her hair is messed up and she appears distressed and sounds very confused.

You talk with her nurse and let her know how confused your aunt is. You also ask if your aunt is on enough pain medication since you have never seen her cry.

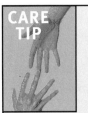

CARE TIP When you enter a patient's room, a special care unit, or even a waiting area, you may need to steel yourself for the unexpected. A hospital is often filled with unfamiliar sights, sounds, and smells. If you are concerned about what you might see, before you go, you may want to ask the patient's nurse about what to expect (presence of IVs, wounds or tubes, state of consciousness).

The family may...

❖ **...find great relief in your presence and want to explain the situation to you.** People often need to repeat, to go over and over what has happened as a way of dealing with the crisis.

❖ **...need to be alone and may be too numb and in shock to say much of anything to you.** Some families pull into themselves during difficult times. It is important to be available to assist, if necessary, but even more important to not intrude on very private family moments.

The visitors may...

❖ **...have gathered.** Some families expect the presence of even very distant relatives in a time of crisis.

❖ **...have come in support.** Some individuals and some families count on folks to surround them during a difficult time. Others may not be ready for this type of attention. Visitors can either be a real comfort to the family or they can be very tiring and distracting.

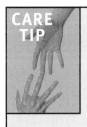

CARE TIP The best thing you can do is check with the family about what will be most helpful. You might want to say, "It looks like this is a family time. I'll be right outside if you need me for anything," or "Would you like me to stay with you or may I go get something for you?"

The hospital world...

Hospitals are foreign to many people. They are like another world. Many folks have never been inside one except when they were born or maybe just to visit someone.

Sorting through the maze...

❖ **The physical layout can seem overwhelming.** It's easy to get turned around.

Anna's story

Your friend Anna was cooking French fries for dinner. When the pan of oil was knocked off the stove, her four-year-old daughter, Lucia, was terribly burned on her face and down the left side of her body. She was rushed to the hospital burn unit.

You arrive to find the waiting room filled with family members. Her parents, Anna and Robert, are at Lucia's bedside. An aunt and Robert's brother, Xavier, have already been on the phone alerting employers and the extended family. Since it's dinnertime, Xavier has taken the lead and has ordered food delivery from a nearby Mexican restaurant.

You sense that Anna's big family is doing okay under the circumstances. Since you've heard that a grandmother will soon be arriving in town by bus, you offer to pick her up and bring her to the hospital.

❖ **It's hard to tell one type of hospital employee from another.** Each hospital has staff from different departments (nursing, medicine, radiology, rehabilitation, lab). And, within each department, employees have different levels of training and experience. For example, within nursing there are usually RNs (registered nurses), LPNs (licensed practical nurses), CNAs (certified nurse aides), etc. Within the medical department, physicians may include medical students, interns, specialists, attending physicians, etc. All of these health-care professionals work together to provide important care for the patients.

❖ **Different units care for patients with different health needs.** Patients are usually assigned to units that care for patients with similar problems.

So, there is the ICU (Intensive Care Unit), CCU (Cardiac Care Unit), NICU (Neonatal Intensive Care Unit), Orthopedic, and Labor and Delivery unit, etc.

❖ **Hospitals have their own language.** You can hear strange terms like PRN, CT Scan, NPO, and I & O. If you are asked to participate in tracking a patient's Intake & Output (I & O), for example, and you don't know what it means, *ask!*

❖ **Health-care workers must protect a patient's privacy.** Due to federal HIPAA (Health Insurance Portability and Accountability Act) regulations, it will likely be very difficult to get details or updates about a patient's condition.

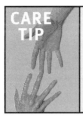

CARE TIP	What you see and hear at the hospital should stay there! If you are a helper, help by maintaining the patient's and the family's privacy. Sharing information will often make life difficult for the patient and family when they resume their normal routine.

Finding your way...

❖ **Correct entrance** In the daytime, this may be the main entrance that has an information desk. At night or on the weekend, the main entrance may be closed and you may be asked to come directly through the emergency room entrance.

❖ **Patient's location** Usually someone at the main entrance or emergency room desk should be able to direct you to the patient's location (room, surgery, Intensive Care Unit). Often, hospitals are like mazes because additions have been put on over the years. You may discover that you need extra help to find your way because you may be upset.

This is common when there's been a crisis. Do not hesitate to ask for help.

❖ **Nurse's station or waiting room** Sometimes a volunteer receptionist is stationed in the waiting room for the Cardiac Care, Intensive Care, or Surgical Care areas. If no one is in the waiting room, find the nurse's station and ask someone to assist you. (The nurse's station is a central work area where nurses and doctors gather to organize patient care.) If you are unsure, ask one of the staff if it's okay for you to see the patient or ask the staff members to let the family know that you have arrived.

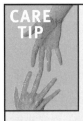

CARE TIP

If you feel anxious or inadequate to deal with what you may find (death, massive injuries, life-threatening diagnosis), you may want to quickly call another person to help you. Choose someone who is both trustworthy and clearheaded and who also knows the family well.

John's story

John rides his bike to work every day. This morning, a driver, blinded momentarily by the morning sun, struck and severely injured John. As his coworker and good friend, you go to the hospital immediately. You head first to the information desk and they tell you to go to the surgical waiting room on the 3rd floor.

Unfortunately, no one is in the waiting room. You look around the hallways and see a hospital worker. The worker directs you to the nursing station down the hall where someone looks up John's whereabouts.

Helping during the hospital stay...

During a hospital stay, family and friends have a unique opportunity to show their caring and concern by tending to very simple and necessary tasks. The smallest effort can make a big difference for an individual and family.

Even a planned hospital stay can be overwhelming. The family's main focus is on the illness or injury. Depending on the severity of the situation and the length of the stay, the family will likely not have the energy to think about their own personal needs or routines at home.

During a hospitalization, the individual's family will probably gather at the hospital. Depending on the situation, the family might need to stay for many hours or even overnight. Parents of a child will often remain nearby throughout the entire stay. So, with all of the stresses on a family, ask yourself what you can do to help make the hospital stay more tolerable.

Paying attention to things at home...

❖ **Has anyone been tending to the needs of the children and any pets?** *Be sure* someone is taking care of them! This can include not only providing supervision and meals (Don't forget the school lunch!), but also taking children to their normal activities (school, lessons, sports, jobs) and helping them to keep in contact with their family during this difficult time.

❖ **Has anyone been taking care of the home?** Someone should pick up mail and newspapers, water the plants, take out the trash, or rotate the lights to keep the home looking lived in. Of course, include family members (if possible) in decisions about the care of the home.

2

Mrs. Henry's story

Eighty-year-old Mrs. Henry was in a car accident on the way home from the grocery store. She was unconscious with severe injuries and was taken by ambulance to the nearest hospital. No one knew until two days later that her only companion, a little terrier, was left alone.

A neighbor heard the dog barking and called the police. Given the situation, the thoughtful neighbor volunteered to take the dog until Mrs. Henry arrived home.

❖ **Is anyone taking messages off the phone?** The family may be awaiting important phone calls that need an immediate response. Always get their permission before taking messages. In some cases, the family may give approval for someone to return calls. Remember to ask for the pin number or password to get into the voicemail messages.

❖ **Is anyone responding to e-mail messages?** In today's world, many people conduct business and correspond with family and friends over the Internet. If you are a trusted friend or family member, you may be asked to simply print off information for the individual's or family's review.

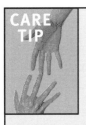

CARE TIP Respect the individual's or family's privacy! Always check with the individual (if his or her condition allows) or family (if they can be contacted) before going into the patient's home to care for children or pets. Ask them for the names of people with whom they feel comfortable caring for their children, pets, and home.

Providing comfort at the hospital...

❖ **Is anyone providing meals for the family in the hospital so family members do not have to leave the patient?** This would allow close family members and friends to gather together in a crisis. Please see "Feeding the body and soul" on page 173.

❖ **Is anyone staying with the patient if family members or very close friends have not yet arrived?** It is not uncommon in emergencies for families to need to travel long distances to get to the bedside of their loved one. If possible, plan for someone to stay with the patient until a family member arrives.

❖ **Is anyone checking with the hospital staff or patient advocate to see if there is a...**

◆ ...recliner or a cot in the patient's room so someone can stay at the bedside.

◆ ...space or locker for family members to keep belongings.

◆ ...place for a family member staying overnight to shower.

◆ ...place for an upset family to have a bit of privacy.

2

Mrs. Chang's story

Mrs. Chang has been rushed to the hospital with signs of a stroke. Amy, her daughter, lives across the country. It will take 18 hours before she can get flight connections and arrive at the hospital.

In the meantime, Amy asks the mother's friend if anyone can stay with her mother or look in on her frequently until she arrives in town. The group of women Mrs. Chang meets with regularly to play cards offers to take turns "being there."

Johnny's story

Nine-year-old Johnny is in critical condition at the hospital after a near drowning. The grandmother is rushed to the hospital to be by his side. In their panic, not only Grandma, but also the entire family has forgotten that Grandma should have taken her medication for diabetes and eaten three hours ago.

A church member asks a close family member about things that they might need from home for the tense overnight stay. He discovers Grandma's problem and immediately goes to the house to get the medication and also something for her to eat.

❖ **Are there special parking arrangements for family and those bringing food and supplies back and forth to the hospital?** Often the hospital will eliminate parking fees or provide parking tokens during a crisis.

❖ **Do the phone calls and visitors need to be limited?** Often numerous calls and visits can upset the individual or family and interfere with the patient's care. Find out how the hospital sets these limits and suggest to the family or nurse that restrictions be considered.

❖ **Has anyone helped the individual or family organize the hospital room?** Hospital rooms are small with little storage or counter space. The room can quickly become cluttered with items that could go home. Supply large sturdy shopping bags or boxes and offer to take the gifts to the family's home.

❖ **Has anyone kept a list of gifts given by well-wishers?** A list can give comfort and a feeling of support, even if the individual or family does not personally respond or acknowledge these gifts. A guest book or "blank book" works great!

Finding hospital resources...

❖ **Do you know someone who works at the hospital** (nurse, physical therapist, respiratory therapist, chaplain, administrator) who might take a special interest in the family and assist if the family has a question or problem? People who work at the hospital can direct you to the right people or resources. They also can help you find your way through the system should a problem arise, or even just visit the individual or family.

❖ **Has a victim's advocate program been contacted to help?** Many states or cities automatically provide assistance to victims of violent crimes or automobile accidents. These advocates can be a tremendous support by providing accurate information during a confusing time and by being a link between various law enforcement groups. They may also help individuals apply for financial, medical, and mental health benefits.

❖ **Should the hospital's social worker or patient advocate be contacted?** These professionals are employed by the hospital to provide assistance to individuals and families. Ask nursing personnel, the information desk receptionist, or the hospital telephone operator for their phone extensions.

These staff members are knowledgeable about patient rights, financial aid, legal issues such as living wills and advance directives, and referrals to community services. They can also help when there is confusion or concern about patient care. In situations requiring financial assistance, the social worker or patient advocate may provide food vouchers, overnight accommodations, transportation, parking tokens, or vouchers.

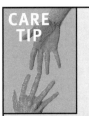

CARE TIP Make a daily list of phone calls and visitors to the hospital. This list can be helpful to the family so they can return calls if they want to. Often, it is not until weeks after a crisis that the individual or family is well enough to review the list of callers. This list can be invaluable in piecing together the events of the past and in building a feeling of support from their community. Supply a pen, guest book, or "blank book" to keep these records.

Bringing a touch of home to the hospital...

❖ **Has anyone offered to retrieve the patient's personal necessities from the home?** If there has not been time to plan for the hospitalization, the patient may not have important personal items (glasses, contact lenses and case, pajamas, hair comb, brush, make-up). *Always* check with the patient or family before searching through the home for personal supplies.

❖ **Has anyone helped the individual or family retrieve comfort items from the home?** Whether the crisis has occurred suddenly or an illness has lasted a long time, the patient (any age) may want comfort items from home. A favorite blanket, pillow, stuffed animal, or photos may provide that comfort as well as a sense of hope, connection to home, and normalcy.

❖ **If someone is staying overnight at the hospital, does he or she have the necessary personal items from home?** See the following checklist that can be used as a reminder before a volunteer either runs home or to the store to get the items.

Personal Items Checklist
For Helpers Staying Overnight

- ☐ Toothbrush
- ☐ Toothpaste
- ☐ Floss
- ☐ Brushes, combs
- ☐ Shampoo
- ☐ Conditioner
- ☐ Deodorant
- ☐ Glasses/case
- ☐ Eye contacts/case
- ☐ Contact lens solution
- ☐ Eye drops
- ☐ Medications
- ☐ Make-up
- ☐ Clean t-shirts
- ☐ Clean pants
- ☐ Change of underwear
- ☐ Socks
- ☐ Shoes
- ☐ Sweaters/sweatshirts
- ☐ More comfortable clothes
- ☐ Pillow
- ☐ Blanket
- ☐ Book
- ☐ Holy book or religious keepsake
- ☐ Special photograph
- ☐ Legal papers (the patient's living will, power of attorney, insurance policies)

2

Being a good visitor...

Visitors to the hospital should come *planning to support* the patient and the immediate family. A worthwhile visit reminds them that they aren't forgotten and brings a moment of relief.

People *should not come* merely to "hang out" and socialize just because many others are visiting. For example, some hospital stays may only last a few days, but are filled with exhausting tests, painful surgery, and tough treatments. For this type of short but intense stay, a visit to the home after the hospital-ization may be more welcomed than a "drop-in" at the hospital.

On the other hand, some lengthier hospital stays may also include difficult procedures, treatments and surgeries, but a visit could very well be a distraction from the illness and bring a welcomed boost. Of course, if someone has very few friends and family, a visit may be "just the ticket."

Coming with a purpose...

❖ **Provide a respite for a family member.** As a close friend, you may be able to stay with the patient while a family member takes a break. This could be for just a few minutes so she or he can take a walk around the hospital or get a cup of coffee. Or, perhaps you could provide a longer break while the family member goes home to nap or freshen up.

> **CARE TIP**
> Years ago, patients were hospitalized for much longer stays. Now, patients are only hospitalized when they are very sick, severely injured, or undergoing intensive procedures. Unless you have been invited, consider staying away at this time. Instead, think about sending your well wishes through the mail, showing your concern by helping in one of the many ways described in this book, or choosing one of your own creation.

❖ **Bring a boost.** A visitor's presence may bring a needed distraction. Both the patient and family members might appreciate a break from the hospital routines and also a connection to the patient's outside world (work, neighborhood, school, social groups).

❖ **Deliver supplies.** The patient or family may need personal items from home or other things to make their stay more tolerable.

Preparing for the unexpected...

❖ **The patient may have pain.** A visitor's presence may be a grateful distraction to some people in pain. For others, however, a visit may only make the pain worse. The patient may need to rest and have "alone time" to lessen the pain, to cope, or to let medication take effect. Visitors should be aware that some patients could carry on conversations without showing obvious signs of pain. Keep your visit short (10-15 minutes) unless specifically asked to stay longer.

❖ **The patient may feel exhausted and need sleep.** Hearing a frightening diagnosis, taking tests, receiving treatments, or enduring a surgery takes a major toll on a person. Most patients have no clue that they are exhausted until after they've had a stream of visitors.

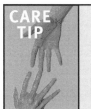
CARE TIP
Though our intentions are good, we all need to be sure that our "helping" is helpful, not harmful. Instead of "dropping in," it is always best to check with the family first for the best time to visit. Be aware that while a family may have said that a particular time might be convenient for a visit, things may have changed. The patient may now need to sleep, cope with pain, or require medical or nursing assistance. Don't be offended if you are asked not to come. Show your concern by helping in one of the many other ways found in this book.

❖ **The patient may feel the need to entertain, but can't and shouldn't.** Patients and family members are often grateful for the support that a visit can show. However, they may feel the need to make the visitor comfortable during a time that is terribly difficult, robbing their energy needed to cope and to heal. Remember, many people will disguise their true feelings, making it difficult to determine if the visit is helpful or harmful. Again, keep your visit to only 10-15 minutes unless specifically asked to stay longer.

❖ **The patient may be nauseated.** Many illnesses, injuries, treatments, or surgeries leave a patient nauseated at intervals.

❖ **The patient may be moody.** Pain, the effects of medication, lack of sleep, and concerns about the illness may keep the patient from being his or her usual self. Stay patient and accepting!

❖ **The patient may be confused or do something out of character.** Medication and illness may also cause the patient to be confused or to say or do something out of character. ***Don't*** take any comments or attitudes personally, and don't tell embarrassing stories about the patient's hospital stay.

❖ **The patient may feel impolite eating a meal in front of visitors.** Patients may not eat when visitors are present, so they won't get the nutrition necessary to regain their health or needed strength. So, avoid visits during mealtimes, excuse yourself when a meal tray arrives, or offer to assist the patient with the meal.

❖ **The patient may have private or urgent needs (go to the bathroom, make a phone call).** A visitor should always remember the hospital room is the patient's only personal space. The patient cannot leave the room to attend to personal needs without everyone knowing, hearing, and smelling. While the visitor may not care, the patient usually does and is very embarrassed! Again, keep your visits short and limited.

❖ **The patient may not remember the visit.** Medication, pain, illness, injury, and a flurry of visitors may cause the patient to forget that you have visited previously.

2

Doris's story

Doris, an elderly woman, was hospitalized after falling and breaking her hip. It has now been two days after her surgery and the room is full of visitors. When the tray arrives, she feels hungry and wants to eat, but hesitates because she's embarrassed to eat in front of everyone.

Her son comes in, sees the full tray of food, and realizes that his mom wants privacy. He asks the nurse to help her get set up for dinner while he takes everyone down to the waiting room for 30 minutes.

Doing something that's helpful...

Always ask yourself, "How can I help?" But, when you come with an idea of how to help, ***be flexible***. It's more important to do what the patient and family would like during the visit rather than to follow your own agenda.

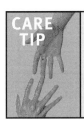

CARE TIP | If you notice that the patient is swamped with visits and is exhausted, consider suggesting that someone posts a sign saying, "No Visitors."

How well you know the patient may also determine what things are appropriate for you to do during your visit. Perhaps the patient may feel comfortable with a very close friend giving a backrub, but not with an acquaintance. Instead, an acquaintance might read a book, play a game, or watch a video with the patient. Make suggestions to the person and see what will work.

For example:

"I brought this book with me. Would you like me to read you a page or two, or would it be better to do it tomorrow?"

"Did you know I love to do people's nails? I've brought my supplies with me. Would you like me to do your nails or is there something else that I can do for you while I'm here?"

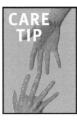

CARE TIP

Always check with the nurses before offering to provide personal care. There may be special precautions due to the individual's health.

Helpful ideas...

❖ Wash the person's hands and apply lotion.

❖ Care for nails (clean, file, apply nail polish).

❖ Wash and set hair.

❖ Assist individual with shaving.

❖ Read a book aloud.

❖ Read faith-based or spiritual passages aloud, checking first to be sure this is okay with the patient.

❖ Quietly sing or hum comforting songs.

❖ Read letters from others aloud.

❖ Assist with feeding and drinking.

❖ Organize the room.

❖ Pray with the individual with his/her approval.

❖ Assist with slow, deep-breathing and relaxation exercises (to help with pain and tension).

❖ Play a game.

❖ Work on a puzzle.

❖ Sit with the person and make an item (knit, sew, draw) to be given to the individual when she or he gets home.

❖ Write letters or notes dictated by the patient.

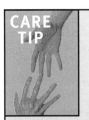

CARE TIP Remember that each day can be very different for the patient, depending on his or her level of pain, fatigue, or condition. Sometimes the patient simply needs to be alone. Sometimes the patient may need the visitor just to listen or to simply sit quietly without making conversation. We don't always have to be doing something to be helpful.

❖   Give back rubs.

❖   Sit quietly.

❖   Watch a video together.

❖   Play an electronic or laptop computer game together.

❖   Share slides/photos of a trip (if you both share a love for traveling).

❖   Listen to music together.

❖   Watch TV together.

❖   Assist with the patient's hobby if he or she is able and if practical in the hospital (getting photos or artwork framed, bringing in hobby supplies).

❖   Create a make-believe trip to the mountains. Bring trail mix, a picnic, sunscreen, water bottle, slides, backpack filled with goodies.

❖   Create a make-believe trip to the ocean. Bring sunscreen, sunglasses, a picnic lunch, sand in bottle, shells, towels, lawn chairs, umbrellas, or CDs of ocean sounds.

❖   Create a make-believe trip to wherever the person dreams of going, complete with props such as music, hats, gear, slides, photos, CDs.

❖   Bring your guitar or other musical instrument and play or sing favorite songs.

❖   Give good old-fashioned hugs.

Alice's story

Alice was hospitalized two days ago after having complications from her chemotherapy treatment. She is very nauseated, exhausted, and unable to eat. To comfort her, Jane, who is in the same book club, reads her a chapter aloud from the book they are currently reading for the next meeting.

2

Note to helpers...

To be sure all of your support is truly kind,
take a look at Chapter 6, "Caring without offending"
and Chapter 7, "What *to* say, what *not* to say."

Now imagine...

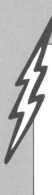

You have just found out that your neighbor is having serious emergency surgery soon. You want to help, but have to go on a business trip. Knowing you have limited time, you decide to stop by the surgical waiting room and bring coffee, bagels, and cream cheese for the anxious relatives. You leave a note for your neighbor, letting him know that you had stopped by, will be going out of town for a week, but will check in with him when you get back.

Or imagine...

You have just found out that your neighbor has had serious emergency surgery. You call to see if the neighbor's husband needs anything. You refer to the checklist on page 41, stop off at the store to pick up the needed items, and find some individually-wrapped snacks to throw in as well.

As you stop by to say hello and drop off the bag of supplies, you ask, "Who is taking care of the pets?" In all the confusion, the husband had totally forgotten about the animals. He gives you a house key so you can feed and care for the pets.

Or imagine this...

You have just found out that your neighbor has had serious emergency surgery with major complications. She is now in the ICU (Intensive Care Unit) in critical condition and her husband is afraid to leave the hospital. You decide to ask other neighbors to join you in helping. Some bring in home-cooked meals, another takes care of the mail and papers, and a neighborhood teenager mows the lawn.

2

CHAPTER THREE

Easing the homecoming...

In this chapter you'll find answers to...

- What challenges does discharge bring?

- How can you get the home ready?

- What can you do to keep the household running?

- How can you make a visit to the home worthwhile?

- What can children do when they visit?

3

Imagine...

Your friend's husband is going home after having been in the hospital for a week and a half. You know that while they are both thrilled that he is finally leaving the hospital, returning home will likely be an exhausting experience. You'd like to help in some way, but don't know what would ease the homecoming.

Coming home from the hospital — the first few weeks...

"You get to go home," used to mean, "You're better." Now, it can just mean that the number of days you are allowed to stay in the hospital is up. Still, most folks long for the time when they can finally go home. But a whole new set of challenges can await them, especially if recuperation will be lengthy or ongoing.

Discharge brings new problems...

❖ The return home will be exhausting. The trauma and the excitement of coming home always take an unexpected toll.

❖ That old cozy bed may now be too low for lifting the patient or providing other care.

❖ The one step at the front door, the narrow doorways, and the tiny bathroom may have turned the house into an obstacle course.

❖ The patient was probably sent home with a fistful of prescriptions that must be filled immediately.

❖ Family members may have to provide difficult treatments and care that previously had been delivered by professionals.

❖ Help will no longer be available at the push of a button any time, day or night. Now, the patient or family member has to navigate through the doctor's office phone system to leave a message and then wait for a call back.

❖ Family members may have to provide care that they do not feel prepared to deliver. They question themselves constantly, "Are we

3

doing it right?" "Are we doing it wrong?" "If we don't do this right, will we hurt our loved one?"

Tweaking the home for easy living...

Homecoming can bring new struggles. Imagine anxiously awaiting the comfort of your home only to find that steps now keep you from going from room to room, the bathroom is now a danger zone with nothing to hold on to, and necessities are out of reach.

Now is when a handyman and even the average person can shine by making the home safe, accessible, and comfortable! Perhaps this is the time people who couldn't help before can jump in to make a difference.

Jobs for the handyman...

❖ **Convert the showerhead to a hand-held shower.** If the patient cannot stand or is weak, a hand-held shower and a shower chair will allow independence.

❖ **Add a tub bar.** Again, this makes getting in and out of the tub safer and easier.

❖ **Add bathroom bars.** Some folks will need bars along the wall for added security.

❖ **Adapt the toilet seat.** Sometimes a raised toilet seat can be attached. Sometimes, a permanent higher toilet will be necessary.

❖ **Build wheelchair ramps.** Inside or out, these ramps make it possible for folks to get around.

> # Bud's story
>
> After the farming accident, Bud will be recuperating in a wheelchair. Bill, his neighbor, knows that Bud will need ramps for his front door and throughout the house.
>
> Bud's friends all want to help, so they pull together the supplies and choose a Saturday to get it all done. By the end of the day, they do a trial run. They ask Bud's wife, Grace, to push Bill in the wheelchair throughout the house to be sure the ramps are strong and the slopes are not too steep.

3

Jobs around the house that anyone can do...

❖ **Rearrange home furniture and living space.** Sometimes this means just moving furniture aside to open up walkways. In other situations, it means moving a bed to the main floor.

❖ **Provide additional lighting.** Sometimes just nightlights throughout will be all that is needed. Other times, additional room lights may be required.

❖ **Put items in reaching distance.** Arrange necessary items close to the bedside so they are easily accessible.

❖ **Remove or stabilize carpets/area rugs.** Throw-rugs are a hazard! Also, area rugs that curl up or can be tripped over should be tacked down with tape or temporarily removed.

❖ **Highlight steps or changes in flooring.** Put brightly-colored tape or lights near steps or a change in levels of flooring.

Common Home Health-Care Needs

☐ Wheelchair
☐ Portable potty or bedpans
☐ Shower or bath chair
☐ Shower or bath bars
☐ Crutches
☐ Reclining chair (A chair in the living room may allow the recuperating family member to be comfortable and still in the midst of things. A recliner can be perfect if the feet need to be up or if the arms need to be supported or steady for IV treatments.)
☐ Towels
☐ Bed sheets

Keeping the household running...

When a family has been hit with a crisis, their focus is on their loved one. The chores around the house likely have been forgotten. When the patient returns home, the family will have so much to do and their energies must go to caring for the sick family member. They will probably need to fill prescriptions, get their loved one comfortable, set up home care, or any number of things.

These days, patients are sent home from the hospital sooner than in years past. So they are much sicker and weaker, requiring more care. Families are often asked to fill in the gap and may need to learn to provide home health care (changing bedpans, giving baths, changing the patient's clothes). They may also need to learn how to change dressings, flush and run IVs, give medications and shots, fill oxygen tanks, or empty urine bags. These new skills can be scary and taking on this responsibility can be upsetting, exhausting, and overwhelming.

Routine household chores would be the last thing on a caregiver's mind. This is a wonderful opportunity for "hands-on" support behind the scenes.

Indoor chores...

Coming home from the hospital with someone who needs to recuperate is hard enough without having to face a mess. No one likes coming home to a mess! If you are close to the patient or family and have gotten the "go-ahead," consider helping with one or more of these chores even before the patient comes home.

❖ **Pick up and organize the mail, papers, or packages.** Even after a week of being gone, the mail has probably piled up. Search for envelopes that look like urgent mail (rent, mortgage, credit card bills, checks). Bring these items to the family's attention immediately. *Never open someone else's mail!*

❖ **Check for old food in refrigerator and put in some fresh.** After getting permission, sort through food in the refrigerator and dispose of spoiled food. Stock the refrigerator with common food items for the patient's homecoming or for out-of-town family members.

❖ **Tidy up the house.** Straighten the house or specific rooms (with the individual's or family's approval only) to ready the house for the patient's homecoming or for out-of-town relatives who arrive and need to stay at the home. Clean the house yourself, get a crew of friends, or pool your money together to hire a cleaning service. *Again, check with the family first!*

❖ **Water the houseplants.** They ought to be thirsty by now!

❖ **Prepare a meal for the homecoming.** The first day home can be so hard and exhausting! Even if the homecoming is exciting, the patient will be ready for a nap. Having a tasty meal waiting could be the best homecoming present ever received. ***Check the patient's diet, allergies, and preferences first!***

❖ **Assist with laundry.** The laundry has just been building up! Again, get approval first, but consider running and folding some loads of non-personal items (sheets, towels, socks, t-shirts, jeans). If you don't know about pre-treating, separating colors, using cold water, and using the delicate cycle, stay away from this task. Leave it for someone who is experienced!

Outdoor chores...

Coming home from the hospital to an overgrown lawn or a snow-packed driveway is so discouraging. With all the things the returning patient will need, the outside chores will be last on the caretaker's list.

❖ **Mow and water the lawn.** This is a great job for a neighborhood teen. Or, you can call a lawn-care service.

❖ **Tend and water the garden or flower boxes.** The first glimpse of a flower or vegetable garden thriving after someone's undergone a difficult health crisis is so encouraging!

❖ **Rake the leaves.** Boy, do they pile up! Again, this is a great way for children and adults to work together to donate their time.

❖ **Shovel the walk or driveway.** A snow-packed or icy driveway or walk can be dangerous. With someone sick at home, getting in and out in an emergency is a must.

❖ **Take out the trash for pickup.** Who wants this building up?

❖ **Walk the dog or care for the critters.** Fido, who has been cooped up while everyone has been at the hospital, would love your attention!

Transportation chores...

If you like to drive cars, getting the family up and running again can be a big help.

❖ **Get the car ready.** If the patient or family has a car, get it ready to be used. Check and fill the tank and tires.

❖ **Drive the patient and caregiver** to medical appointments, therapies, etc.

❖ **Pick up prescriptions or supplies.** Usually a patient leaves the hospital with a handful of prescriptions, including painkillers, that must be filled right away. Plan to have someone ready and able to do this even before the patient leaves the hospital, if possible.

❖ **Take children to their activities** (school, church, lessons, sport practices, events, etc.) This job should only be for someone the family totally trusts. *Get permission first!*

❖ **Pick up visiting relatives** from the airport, train, or bus station.

3

Judy's story

Betty offers to make a run to the pharmacy to get medication for Judy, who is coming home from the hospital today. When she delivers the package to Judy's husband, he invites her to stay and visit. Knowing that Judy will be exhausted just from the homecoming, Betty declines the invitation, promising to visit her later in the week when things have settled down.

Making your visit memorable...

Be sure your visit helps, not hinders! Most visits should last only 15–20 minutes. If you're coming to give the caregiver a break, it can be longer. Make your time count!

"A bit personal" visit ideas...

Attach a bit of comfort to your visit! The list below can give you ideas for things to do when visiting. However, check first, because what's okay for one might be too private for another. For instance, one person might just love having polish put on her toenails. Another might be embarrassed because she doesn't like having her toes touched or doesn't like anyone seeing the condition of her feet.

For example, you might want to say, " I'm able to visit this afternoon. Would you like me to bring supplies to give you a manicure, wash your hair, or just bring a movie that we can watch together?"

❖ **Wash the patient's hands.** This simple act is often forgotten and difficult for someone in bed to do. The smell of soap and really clean hands after a hospital stay can be refreshing.

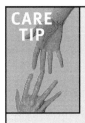

CARE TIP

Visit with the goal of helping out. Don't expect to be fed or entertained! Unless you are sitting with the patient at the caretaker's request (for a short nap or to run an errand), keep your visit short and stay focused on the task at hand. After you're done, leave.

❖ **Apply lotion** to dry hands and feet or arms and legs.

❖ **Give a backrub.** A light touch is important! Not everyone would be comfortable with this, so ask first.

❖ **Groom fingernails or toenails.** Be sure to check first. Sometimes, an individual's health (diabetes) may require special precautions or that nail care be done in a doctor's office.

❖ **Paint fingernails, toenails.** Sometimes this is even amusing for boys or men, especially if the individual has a leg cast or an arm cast.

❖ **Clean up, pick up, and organize things.** Be sure to get an okay first from the individual or family, but a little tidying-up in the patient's room or kitchen, etc., can be a pick-me-up!

❖ **Wash or do hair.** Ahhh! What could be better than getting your hair cleaned after being in bed for a week or two or three! This can be tricky, however, if the person is still bedridden, so plan ahead.

❖ **Spend the evening or the night.** Having an extra person in the house to listen for the patient's calls for assistance gives the exhausted caregiver a break. What a gift!

3

Lucia's story

After being terribly burned, multiple life-saving surgeries have left Lucia very scarred. Consumed with grief and shock, her mom, Anna, is sometimes overwhelmed by the many folks who have come to the home to offer loving support.

As her friend, you have been helping to keep the house running by doing the laundry and fixing simple meals whenever you can. Knowing that the constant stream of visitors has sometimes exhausted Anna, you and Anna come up with a plan. She will pull on her left ear to signal you when she needs some rest. When you see the signal, you will kindly finish up the conversations and show the well-wishers to the door.

❖ **Just listen.** Sometimes just being a listening ear for either the patient's or the caregiver's thoughts and feelings can provide a welcomed relief. As a visitor it is important to know when to be quiet. You don't need to have the answers or to give advice unless asked.

❖ **Take care of the children.** If you are a trusted friend of the family, consider entertaining the children for a morning, an evening, or a night.

"Less personal" visit ideas...

Let's say you want to make your visit count, but you don't know the person well. What can you do? Try some of these things. Again, give the person or the caretaker a choice.

Easing the homecoming...   65

For example, try saying, "I know you like sports and I just read a terrific magazine article I could read to you." Or, "My handwriting isn't bad. If you would like me to write some letters or e-mails for you, I could. What can I help you with when I come to visit this afternoon?"

Dwayne's story

Joyce delivered a home-cooked meal to Dwayne's family. Dwayne, who is quite elderly, has been dealing with multiple illnesses and is now in his last month of life. Joyce had planned to zip in and out since Dwayne had just gotten back from getting transfusions at the hospital and she knew he needed to rest. In addition, extended family members from out of town had just arrived.

When Selma, Dwayne's wife, walked Joyce out to the kitchen, she began to sob and shared that she had just heard that Dwayne's chemo treatments were no longer working and would be stopped. The doctor had told Selma this morning that Dwayne was not expected to live much longer. All hope had been ripped away from her. Joyce hugged her, just listened, and let Selma cry. When Joyce left, she realized that her gift of the meal was far less important than her gift of listening.

3

❖ **Read aloud or listen to "talking books" together.** Share an article or read a book of the individual's choice. If you can visit on an ongoing basis, consider reading a bit each visit. It will give the patient something to look forward to.

❖ **Read religious passages** if they are comforting to the patient.

❖ **Listen to music together,** especially, if you both share a love for a particular type of music.

❖ **Sing or hum songs.** Maybe the patient will join in and you can both enjoy an old-fashioned sing-along.

❖ **Bring and read letters** sent from groups the person belongs to (school, neighborhood, work, church, sports clubs).

❖ **Fix a meal.** If the patient can be up and about or can sit in a chair, consider having your visit in the kitchen while you are preparing a tasty treat. The two of you can chat! (See "Feeding the body and soul" on page 165 for more ideas.)

❖ **Bring a piece of cake** (or other treat) to eat *with* the person. Sometimes it's the conversation that comes *with the treat* that makes a difference.

❖ **Handwrite notes and cards** for the patient who is too weak to do it alone. Be the secretary and help the patient stay in touch with friends and family.

❖ **Go for a walk and get a breath of fresh air.** If the patient is in a wheelchair, go for a spin. Be sure to ask what activity restrictions were given at discharge.

❖ **Sit on the porch.** Sometimes, just a bit of sun and new scenery makes all the difference!

Visiting ideas for children...

If invited, well-behaved children can bring happiness and diversion to a person or family struggling with illness. Be sure to keep the visit short

(5 - 10 minutes) and be aware of the patient's condition. As adorable as children might be, people who have loved to see them in the past may be too exhausted and sick to see them now. And, remember, most people try to put up a good front, so don't wait to leave until they are obviously irritated, tired, or in pain.

It's important for children to actively show that they care. Any of these ideas are positive ways to make their visit count.

❖ **Make and share a card or picture.** Give a child some crayons and paper and "Shazaam!" A masterpiece will appear! Even the smallest child will proudly deliver a homemade creation that will bring smiles.

❖ **Write and share a story or poem.** This is a great way for older children to show they care.

❖ **Make and bring a small gift.** For ideas for making a gift, see the "Giving the perfect gift" on page 195.

❖ **Make and deliver a book of letters and photos or a video of well-wishes from neighbors.** Neighborhood kids can work together on this project. It not only keeps them busy but also gives them a great way to show their concern.

❖ **Read a story.** This is a great way for an older child to entertain a younger sick child.

❖ **Bring homemade cookies, muffins, or cupcakes.** Check first to see that these sweets are okay for the patient. Find kid-friendly recipes. Be sure an adult supervises if the use of an oven is necessary.

❖ **Care for the home critters.** The pets need to be fed, watered, and exercised day in and day out. And, no matter what, the cages or aquariums can always use a cleaning. This can be a perfect way for an older child to help. ***Be sure that they get permission first!***

❖ **Pray.** This is something that any child of any age of any faith can do.

❖ **Do outdoor chores.** Imagine how wonderful it would be for an older child to visit and to volunteer to do a job. Children can water plants, mow the lawn, rake leaves, shovel snow, or take out the trash. It's essential that young people learn to give without expecting money in return!

Mr. Thompson's story

Eleven-year-old Billy wanted to visit his elderly neighbor, Mr. Thompson, who had come home from the hospital. After two weeks, Mr. Thompson's lawn badly needed mowing. Billy's mom suggested that he help by mowing the lawn and then by stopping in to visit for a couple of moments. She reminded him that Mr. Thompson would try to pay him, but that he should plan to say, "No, the best pay you can give me is to get better!" Billy came home feeling really good knowing that he had done something really special.

Note to helpers...
To be sure all of your support is truly kind,
take a look at Chapter 6, "Caring without offending"
and Chapter 7, "What ***to*** say, what ***not*** to say."

Now imagine...

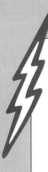

Your close friend has been at her husband's side over the last two weeks after a surgery that had many complications. When you go by to water the plants one last time before they come home, you notice that the refrigerator is full of old moldy food. You decide to clean it out and put in some fresh milk, bread, eggs, and fruit to tide them over.

3

Or imagine...

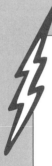

You know that your friend from church will be overwhelmed with caring for her 10-year-old daughter, Molly, who is coming home from the hospital's burn center tomorrow. Molly will need constant attention for her severe burns and her continuing recovery.

In the midst of this, your friend is worried about how her other two children will get to their activities. You offer to drive the two children to their music lessons and tutoring sessions for the next several weeks. Mom gladly accepts your offer.

Or imagine this...

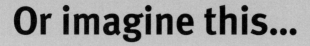

After John's debilitating stroke, you rally a bunch of his buddies from work to make his bathroom in his one-level home more handicapped-accessible. With careful planning, everyone has a task and will bring the necessary tools and materials.

You bring doughnuts and coffee to the Saturday work morning to get everyone going. The workers meet at John's house with the goal of equipping the bathroom with a hand-held shower, shower chair, built-in bathroom bars, and a new toilet designed for the handicapped. Because of the many hands working together, the job was done by noon.

Your coworker comes home, grateful for his friends' help. With a safe bathroom, some assistance, and continued rehabilitation, he will be able to become more independent.

CHAPTER FOUR

Helping over the long haul...

In this chapter you'll find answers to...

- How do different long-term illnesses progress as time goes on?

- How can you make a visit to the home count?

- How do you know if your help is too much or not enough?

4

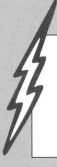

Imagine...

Your coworker will need continual care at home for a very
long time following a bad car accident. Your time is limited,
but you would like to visit and help your friend somehow.

Matching your help to the situation...

Illnesses can take several different forms. Sometimes the patient's condition gets worse. Sometimes the condition gets worse off and on. Some will never improve. Adjust the amount and type of help you give to fit the needs of the situation. The diagrams below give a picture of each type of condition.

The condition that gets better with time...

After an initial health crisis, the patient steadily improves, regaining the strength needed to get around and to return to previous activities.

EXAMPLES: heart attack, mild stroke, injury, surgery (joint replacement, appendix, eye)

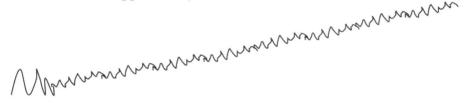

4

David's story

After putting up with a bad knee for some time, David, a 42-year-old plumber, decided to finally have a knee replacement. Because he has lived alone for a long time, his coworkers decide to take turns bringing in meals once David gets home. His neighbors promise to pick up the mail and bring in the newspapers for as long as he needs it.

His two best buddies will alternate coming to the house every day, to make sure that David does all of the exercises and walking he's supposed to do to get back to normal.

The condition that only gets worse with each episode...

After an initial health crisis, the patient has continuing setbacks. With each setback, his or her condition gradually worsens.

EXAMPLES: a series of strokes, heart attacks, or permanent damage from an accident with continuing complications

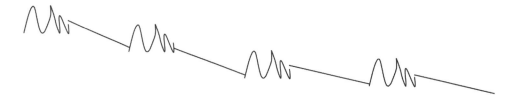

Bessie's story

Bessie has had one stroke after another. The strokes have affected her ability to swallow, her speech, her balance, and her ability to walk by herself. With each stroke, she has lost more independence.

Her church friends have stuck with her through thick and thin. Some take her to rehabilitation while others always cook a little extra and package up frozen meals for her. The church youth take turns mowing her lawn and shoveling her walk throughout the year. Family members help her with day-to-day personal hygiene and dressing.

The condition that gets worse off and on...

After the initial health crisis, the patient endures a number of setbacks, ongoing surgeries, and treatments. Even though the patient struggles off and on, he or she remains stable.

> **EXAMPLES:** a series of cancer treatments, severe epilepsy, ongoing surgeries, or intermittent burn treatments

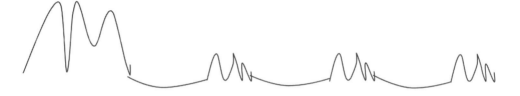

Jill's story

Jill, a three-year-old child, was rescued from a terrible fire, but suffered severe burns to her face and the left side of her body. Every so often, she must return to the hospital for additional painful surgeries and physical therapy.

The family leaves the six-year-old brother with the aunt's family, who live several miles away. Neighbors help by collecting the mail and the papers, and by watering the flowers around the family's mobile home. The older neighborhood kids take turns caring for the guinea pig and the fish.

4

The condition that gradually but steadily gets worse...

The patient's symptoms gradually increase and the person's overall condition worsens over time.

EXAMPLES: Alzheimer's disease, Lou Gehrig's disease, emphysema, aging

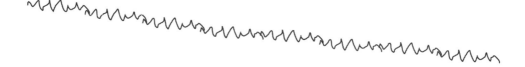

Terry's story

Terry is only 60, but has been diagnosed with Alzheimer's disease. For the moment, he and his wife, Mary, are able to stay in their apartment with the help of some of their friends, neighbors, and relatives.

Since Terry must have someone with him all the time, the retired couple next door helps by either running simple errands or staying with Terry when Mary goes out. As Terry's condition worsens, friends come in more often to either take Mary out or just provide her with company. Ralph, Terry's brother, comes by twice a week to help Terry take a shower.

The condition that rapidly gets worse...

The patient's illness begins suddenly and the patient's condition quickly declines.

EXAMPLES: some quickly spreading and untreatable cancers, deadly infections

4

Ruth's story

Ruth is only 52, but has gotten a terrible case of pneumonia and is not improving despite intensive hospital care. Her only sister has been notified and is coming into town. Two of her coworkers keep in touch with the hospital and take turns stopping by the apartment to feed the cat.

Sadly, Ruth dies. After the service in Ruth's hometown, the two coworkers help the sister pack up Ruth's belongings and clean up the apartment. One of the coworkers finds a home for the cat.

The condition that stays the same...

This type of condition can happen in different ways. For example, after a significant health crisis, the person never fully recovers, but his or her situation remains stable, yet needs continual support.

EXAMPLES: permanent damage from a head or spinal cord injury, severe genetic disorder, debilitating stoke

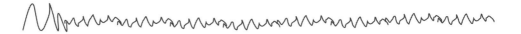

At home support—make your visit count!

When most people visit someone at home who is sick or injured, they see it as a time to sit and talk. Sometimes, a friendly chat may be exactly what's needed. However, when someone is facing a lengthy illness or recovery, consider making your visit even more useful.

Think about making your next visit memorable for the patient by combining chatting with some sort of activity. Often it's easier and more comfortable for everyone to chat while doing something else rather than just having a conversation. Imagine how wonderful it could be for the patient if a visitor planned to play a game, watch TV, or go for a walk together.

Or, consider what a relief it would be for the caregiver if the visitor provided some practical help. Give a giant gift by offering to do chores, by letting the caregiver take a quick break, or by teaching family members basic living skills that the patient can no longer do.

Paul's story

Paul, a young accountant, was on his way up the corporate ladder. He was an avid biker, but one weekend, a car hit him, leaving him with numerous injuries and permanent brain damage.

Even after months of rehabilitation, he is still unable to work or drive. Because he needs continual help just remembering the simplest things, Paul has had to move back in with his family. His world has suddenly become very small.

Friends from work occasionally take Paul out and they try to include him in some company events. But he is not the same old Paul. Now, he tends to get very emotional without warning. He recognizes that he has changed a lot and worries that he will always be dependent on others.

Al, a fellow biker, feels terrible for his friend and knows the same thing could have easily happened to him. Because of this, he decides to hang in there with Paul "over the long haul" and visit every Thursday night.

He chats with Paul's parents, learns about Paul's rehabilitation goals and gets hints on how to help Paul when he gets upset. On most Thursday nights, Al and Paul grab some "fast food," watch TV, or walk around the lake. Paul's parents can now count on a few hours each week to get away together.

4

Spending time with the patient...

Sometimes seeing a fresh face when you are homebound is not only a relief to the patient, but to the caregiver as well. Upbeat visitors can bring activity and laughter into the home.

❖ **Eat lunch together.** Either bring along a special meal or prepare something there at the home. If you have a special treat in mind, bring along the necessary ingredients and the recipe so you are prepared.

Bobby's story

Grandma knows that her grandson loves a special meal from a nearby restaurant. Bobby is homebound for three months during chemotherapy. Each time she visits she brings his favorite takeout meal and they both have lunch together while they watch Bobby's favorite TV show.

❖ **Clean or style hair.** Someone who's good with washing, cutting, and styling hair could really make a difference here! Just a reminder, medical supply stores or pharmacies may have helpful equipment to make washing the bedridden person's hair easier.

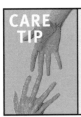

CARE TIP

Doing something together can break the uncomfortable tension of needing to make conversation.

❖ **Play a game.** Any favorite game will do! If you meet on a frequent basis, have an ongoing checkers or card game competition. This can give the homebound person something to look forward to.

❖ **Watch TV.** Perhaps the visitor arrives while the sick person is watching a favorite TV program. Instead of turning off the program, the visitor can offer to watch the TV show as well. Be sensitive to the fact that a TV show may be one of the patient's highlights for the week.

❖ **Watch a movie.** Bring a movie with you to share or find out the patient's favorite flick. Consider the person's age, family/individual values, and the content and tone of the movie. A sad movie that includes death and illness may be upsetting at this time.

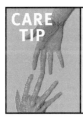 **CARE TIP** To be helpful, your visit should work around the homebound person's schedule as much as possible. Even if someone is homebound, he or she likely has a plan for the day.

❖ **Read aloud.** Sometimes the comforting sound of a friend or relative's voice can distract from pain and boredom. Reading may lull someone in pain to sleep or break up the monotony of the day.

❖ **Listen to music.** Music can connect people and can help break through awkward moments. For a teenager who is nervous about visiting a sick friend, sharing music might cut through the tension. And, for a really sick kid, listening to the latest "hit" is a good way to feel like he or she is still "in the loop."

❖ **Just listen.** Often, a listening ear is the best medicine. Perhaps the patient does not want to burden his or her caregiver with woes and complaints. Or, perhaps the family is exhausted and just needs a break.

❖ **Go for a walk.** A bit of fresh air is great for anyone, weather permitting! A stroll (even if the person is in a wheelchair) around the apartment complex or neighborhood provides a great change of scenery and often a chance to say "hi" to neighbors.

4

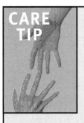

CARE TIP

Sometimes it's helpful to share a similar experience, if you have one, to show that you understand the issues. This does not mean "one-upping." It won't make the person or family feel better if you say, "Well, if you think you have it bad, you should hear what happened to me!"

On the other hand, it could bring comfort if someone knows that "you've been there." If you have had a *very* similar experience (your child has *also* suffered from X disease, your father has ALSO developed Alzheimer's, you've *also* been diagnosed with cancer), then let the person know *without* going into detail.

Helping the other family members...

When someone is sick, other family members still need to continue on with their lives. Children need to get to school or their activities. Elderly adults living in the home may still need to get to church, to a job, or see friends.

❖ **Give the caregiver time away.** The day in and day out grind of providing care to a loved one can be exhausting. Sometimes a friend can spontaneously offer the caregiver an hour or two away. Other times, someone can commit to a set time each week. Or, perhaps a group can be put together and each person can take turns every week offering respite care.

❖ **Watch the children.** Just taking the children for a short time or going on an outing provides a getaway for the kids and a break for the parents. If possible, offer to care for the children on a regular basis. For example, perhaps take the children every Thursday afternoon after soccer practice or have them come over every Saturday morning.

Ned's story

Ned knows that his cousin will take over the care for his wife every Thursday afternoon. Ned uses this time to go out with friends, go fishing, go to the movie theater, or anything to relax. Even if it has been a rough week, he looks forward to his Thursday afternoons just for himself.

❖ **Spend time with other family members.** Perhaps there are other adult family members who also rely on the family caregiver to get to appointments or to run errands. Now the caregiver must focus solely on the sick person and cannot assist the other loved one. Think about taking out this elderly grandparent or relative needing attention.

Danny's story

Danny, a 15 year old, is recovering from a bone marrow transplant. Though his sister, Dylan, is attending college across the country, she is able to fly home and visit every weekend thanks to some generous folks. These special individuals have turned in their frequent flyer miles in exchange for Dylan's plane tickets. Danny looks forward to the upbeat connection that only his sister can provide.

4

Assisting with the household chores...

Families exhausted by worry and the constant (and sometimes intense) care of a loved one are often not able to tend to household chores. Jumping in to tackle some of the routine tasks can be a tangible gift of friendship and support.

❖ **Do the laundry.** Consider running a few loads of laundry while you're at the house. Some families/individuals, however, may be very uncomfortable with anyone sorting their laundry. On the other hand, they might be okay with someone washing specific piles, such as the towels, bed linens, etc. *Ask first!*

❖ **Take out the trash.** This is something that always has to be done, but rarely would anyone ask you to do it. So an offer to collect the trash and then take it to the outside trash can, trash bin, or curb could be very welcomed. Find out how they want it done.

❖ **Cook.** Once a month or so, think about fixing the person's/family's favorite meal or dish. This special treat will give everyone something to anticipate.

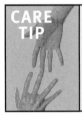

CARE TIP

Consider pulling a number of people together to help with periodic cooking, cleaning, or laundry.

❖ **Clean.** While you are giving a family member a break, tidy up the bedroom and bathroom. If the individual is taking a nap and can be left alone, pick up the nearby living area or kitchen, too.

❖ **Organize the refrigerator.** This may seem an impossible task for the individual or family just trying to cope. Pack up recent leftovers for individual frozen entrees, throw out spoiled food, and clean the refrigerator. *Ask first!*

❖ **Organize the medical reports, bills, or insurance forms.** The never-ending delivery of medical bills and insurance forms can overwhelm and confuse the struggling caregiver. Come in once a week or so to review, organize, and file the documents.

❖ **Help with the family pets.** Maybe the family is able to feed and care for the pet, but unable to exercise the animal or clean the cages. Offer to do these more time-consuming jobs when needed.

❖ **Do yard work.** When an illness is at its peak, a family may not be able to water, mow the lawn, or rake the leaves. Provide some welcomed relief by picking up the slack.

❖ **Tend the garden.** Often people plant a garden with great hopes for the harvest, but then, due to illness, are not able to keep it up. Weeding, watering, picking, and preparing the vegetables for the individual or family would be a wonderful, nutritious gift.

❖ **Shovel the snow.** Imagine being stranded and unable to get out of the driveway or road when you are worrying that you might have to go to the hospital or get needed supplies. Relieve an anxious mind by shoveling or plowing away the snow and ice.

4

❖ **Run errands.** Offer to run the errand or perhaps stay with the ill person while the caregiver goes. Sometimes even the mundane job of filling a prescription or going to the dry cleaners can be a refreshing break for someone stuck at home.

❖ **Pick up groceries.** Letting a family know that you go to the grocery store every Saturday morning and that you can always pick up a few extra items can be helpful. Or, you can offer to go to the grocery and fill their list once a week. Maybe a group of willing folks can be organized to take turns.

Helping other family members learn new skills...

With a chronic illness, traditional family roles often shift. The husband may need to do more of the cooking or the wife may need to attend to financial matters. Or, perhaps the older child may need to provide more care for the younger children. These changes will take time and will sometimes be painful to watch. An encouraging and patient person can help here by sharing his or her knowledge and experience.

❖ **Grocery shopping** Grocery shopping is an essential part of keeping the household running. While some folks will never love to shop or learn the art of saving with coupons, they should learn the basics of watching for expiration dates on containers, picking good produce, and saving money by shopping for "best buys."

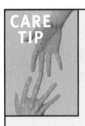

CARE TIP Every household's routines are different. Some clean more than others. Some use only fresh fruits and vegetables, while some only use frozen or canned. Some household routines are relaxed while others are tightly scheduled. Be sure to respect each family's way of life.

❖ **Preparing meals** Find out about the family's eating patterns. What kinds of foods does the family eat? Do they eat a large meal at lunch or at dinner, or do they simply snack throughout the day? Locate the family's cookbook or favorite recipes if they have them. Consider getting a cookbook for them that requires only a few ingredients.

As easy as it may seem, some folks may not even know how to use a microwave oven. Find out who will now be helping with the cooking and how much the new cook has been in the kitchen in the past. Start with a simple and favorite recipe. Just be the guide, letting the new cook do the cooking.

❖ **Cleaning the home** The never-ending chore! Do family members know where the cleaning equipment is and how to use it? Do they know what needs to be done and when? Do they know how to run the vacuum?

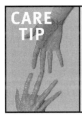

CARE TIP

Perhaps you can only be available to help for a week, a month, or every now and then. ***Be careful not to promise help that you cannot deliver.***

❖ **Washing dishes** Someone has to do them! Be sure someone is learning how to do this. You may need to give several lessons on this.

❖ **Running the laundry** A lot of clothes can pile up in a hurry. Show someone in the family how to separate the clothes by colors, use the washing machine and dryer, wash by temperature, measure laundry soap, pre-treat for stains, fold clothes, and put them away.

❖ **Maintaining the car** Many people have never had to maintain a car or even fill it with gas. If this is a new responsibility, consider offering to go with them to the service station to help them learn the basics.

◆ **Fill the tank.** Be sure he or she can remove the gas cap. This is sometimes hard for those with arthritic hands. At many gas stations you can pay either at the pump or at the counter. Walk them through paying both ways until they feel confident.

4

- ◆ **Put air in the tires.** Checking the tires for air is important for both safety and the life of the tires. Be sure to show how to check the car manual or tire specifications for the correct air pressure (PSI) that is needed.

- ◆ **Change a flat tire.** Hopefully no one will have to do this, but everyone should be prepared. Show the person where to find the spare tire, the jack, and the car manual.

- ◆ **Check and change the oil.** A family enduring a chronic illness does not need the car to break down! But if the person who maintained the car is now unable, other family members may need to learn how this is done.

- ◆ **Heed warning lights.** Overwhelmed family members may be tempted to ignore warning lights. They may not even understand the meaning of the lights or the importance of getting help immediately when they come on. This again is a good opportunity to show how to use the car manual and where to get service.

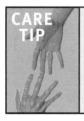

CARE TIP

While it might be easy for some, learning how to maintain a car may be overwhelming for others.

- ❖ **Finances** Is anyone remembering to pay the bills? Perhaps the person who is now laid up used to pay all the bills, balance the checkbook, or track the bank statements. Teaching someone to do this can be invaluable.

❖ **Insurance** Along with an illness comes a flood of insurance papers and bills. Organizing these forms can be a nightmare! Check to be sure someone knows how to deal with this task.

❖ **Disability Insurance/Social Security Disability** When someone has a catastrophic illness or accident, he or she may qualify for some type of disability insurance. Having someone sort out this maze and explain what needs to be done can be such a gift.

❖ **Ongoing homecare** Without experience, it's often difficult to know if your loved one is receiving quality care. When ongoing professional home care (nursing, respiratory, physical therapy) is necessary, a friend in the health field may help you find quality care and show you what to watch for.

❖ **Organizing medications** Taking the right amount of medication at the right time can be critical. Show the patient or a family member how to organize, pack, or prepare the medications for the week. Double check each week until you're sure they've got it!

❖ **Rehabilitation exercises** Become familiar with the rehabilitation exercises given by the therapist. Then, think about visiting on a regular basis and encourage the person to exercise while you are there.

❖ **Treatment options** People enduring a chronic illness are often looking for better solutions. They may want to research their condition, find new drugs or new ways to help with pain, explore better treatments, or enter experimental treatment programs. Someone with library or Internet searching skills might be able to help here.

❖ **Taxes** Taxes wait for no one! You may need to coach a family member through this process. You may also need to design a file system to keep future receipts, statements, and other papers organized for the next year's taxes.

❖ **Chauffeuring** Find out about the weekly schedule. Do family members need to get to school, lessons, church activities, or sporting events? You may be able to help by making a schedule or writing (or even drawing) directions.

❖ **Legal issues** Sometimes an accident leaves the individual or family with legal issues. Most will need help wading through the legal system and process. Someone who has both professional legal experience and the family's best welfare in mind can be helpful here.

❖ **Job search** Sometimes an illness or an accident leads you down a new path. Are you a friend who has good job connections or knows how to write a resume? Maybe you are good at identifying someone's strengths or interests that could lead to a new career. Sharing this talent with someone who is struggling with a chronic illness could jumpstart his or her new life.

Being there long term — fostering independence...

Initially, the individual or family in crisis may need a lot of assistance. However, there's a fine line between lending *enough support* and giving *too much.* Lending enough support helps people learn the skills they will need to eventually handle things on their own. On the other hand, giving too much robs them of the opportunity to learn how to care for themselves.

Swooping in to lift up an individual or family for a week or two is very different than smothering them constantly with too much help "over the long haul."

When bad things happen, most people will want to reach out to help and that's really good. But when an individual or family is enduring long-term or permanent changes (loss of a young mother or father, loss of a spouse, getting a major disability), they will need some "alone time" to sort things out, to begin to cope on their own, and to build a new life.

Provide support without taking over and without intruding. It's important for people to believe that they can help themselves because that is how they heal, develop hope, and take pride in new responsibilities.

For example, immediately after a crisis, a family may need help with meals or with arranging transportation to medical appointments. However, as things begin to settle down, they likely can and should be encouraged to start doing these things on their own.

Slowly, cut back on your help and do just enough to help the individual or family get on their feet. The goal is not to fix everything or take away every bit of life's pain, but to help people rebuild their lives.

4

Note to helpers...
To be sure all of your support is truly kind,
take a look at Chapter 6, "Caring without offending"
and Chapter 7, "What *to* say, what *not* to say."

Now imagine...

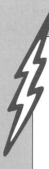

You stop by to visit your coworker who is in the middle of a long recuperation following a terrible car accident. You encourage his mother, who has been staying with him, to take a break while you are there. After getting instructions about his diet, you fix a simple lunch for the two of you to share.

Or imagine...

Knowing that your coworker's mother is getting exhausted by the long-term care her son requires, you offer to visit every other Saturday morning to give her some time away. While you visit with your friend, you wash the dishes in the sink and tidy up the room.

Or imagine this...

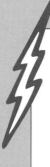

During your coworker's long rehabilitation, you find other folks from work who are interested in helping. Following a weekly schedule, they mow the lawn, run errands and clean the house.

CHAPTER FIVE

Comforting the grieving...

In this chapter you'll find answers to...

- What's life like for folks who have lost a loved one?

- What are some common gifts people give when someone dies?

- How can you help when someone has just died?

- What can you do to help with the service or reception?

- How can you help as time goes by?

5

Imagine...

Your daughter's ballet teacher died after a very short illness. You've sent a sympathy card, but you'd like to do more to help.

What it's like for people who are grieving...

The faces of grief are often surprising. Because of shock and the resulting protective numbness after a death, outward signs of grief may not occur immediately. As the numbness wears off, the grief-stricken may become more keenly aware of their loss and express their grief more intensely.

People in grief may appear...

❖   ...as if nothing has happened.

❖   ...totally devastated.

❖   ...weary.

❖   ...driven.

❖   ...unconcerned.

❖   ...overly concerned.

❖   ...anxious or restless.

❖   ...calm.

❖   ...reckless (drinking, using drugs).

❖   ...lonely.

People in grief may mourn for the loss of...

❖   ...someone who can laugh, cry, share stories, or talk about intimate issues and concerns.

5

❖   ...someone to share a bed with.

❖   ...having someone around all of the time.

❖   ...dreams for future birthdays, school days, graduations, marriage, children, grandchildren.

❖   ...common milestones (1st smile, 1st words, 1st steps, 1st day of school)

❖   ...someone to pass on a family name, family traits, and the family line.

❖   ...a parent who knew their history and cared about them.

People in grief may feel...

❖   ...hopeless and disinterested in life.

❖   ...numb and unaware of surroundings.

❖   ...empty because of losing dreams, hopes, and beliefs about life.

❖   ...afraid because of being blind-sided, hurt by life, and shaken when beliefs have been destroyed.

❖   ...out of control and panicky, feeling as if she or he is falling apart.

❖   ...confused about life's rules. What used to work suddenly may not.

❖   ...overwhelmed because he or she may not know what to do or which way to turn.

❖ ...paralyzed. Very capable people may suddenly be unable to concentrate enough to complete even the simplest tasks or make the simplest decisions.

❖ ...isolated perhaps due to being avoided or forgotten by others. This can occur even with a spouse present if she or he cannot support the other or cannot accept support.

❖ ...different because life is now out-of-the-ordinary and he or she cannot fit into the mold of "normal."

❖ ...changed and may seem unfamiliar even to himself or herself.

❖ ...empty as if there is nothing left inside.

❖ ...physically ill including having aches and pains, nausea, dizziness, heaviness in the chest, fatigue, poor appetite, or insomnia. Remember, any physical symptoms should not be ignored or assumed to be just the result of grief. Get a check-up!

❖ ...angry at the deceased or at God.

Grief has its own timeline...

A survivor *may* or may *not*...

❖ **...return to a previous routine.** Some may return immediately, some take weeks, months, or years, and some may never resume their previous life's activities.

❖ **...seek professional counseling.** Counseling may be helpful immediately, later, or never.

5

❖   **...find support in the people around them.** While some may reach out to those around them, others may want to leave their friends and family to make a "new start."

❖   **...find comfort in organized support groups.** Some folks may be able to connect with people who share similar experiences. Others might not want to join, fearful that by listening to someone else's story, they would add to their own pain. Some might seek organized group support later on. Support groups can be found in many different places (churches, funeral homes, hospice centers, hospitals, police headquarters.) Check with the individual organization or find lists in the library, in the local newspaper, or on the Internet.

❖   **...find comfort from an individual who has shared a similar experience.** Some may find help from just one trusted acquaintance instead of sharing in a large group setting.

❖   **...glean comfort from books or movies.** Some learn better about the grieving process from the safe distance of a book or movie.

Reminders for helpers...

❖   **Don't impose grieving timelines or expectations.** Just because you or someone you know "moved on" in one year, does not mean everyone should or could. Comparing one person's experience of grief to another's assumes that there is only one right way to grieve.

❖   **Don't encourage the survivor to make any major decisions immediately.** Remember, a death often brings intense feelings, causing people to feel the need to move, change jobs, or even sever ties with family or friends. Once the initial shock and numbness has worn off, a person may regret having made radical changes.

❖ **Don't impose your own loss experience on others.** Just because your loving parent died does not mean the other person lost a parent he or she felt close to. Perhaps his parent was not loving or kind.

❖ **Don't think people will "get over" their loss.** Hopefully, they will find a way to "move on" with their grief.

❖ **Remember that new situations, everyday happenings, or special occasions may trigger intense emotion.** This can happen even years after the loss.

❖ **Realize that each person is trying to find his or her own path back to living.** It is important to support whatever path he or she takes. You can't "fix things" for them or cheer them up, and lecturing or scolding won't speed up the grieving process.

❖ **And, finally, remember that as milestones come up, the survivor may struggle more emotionally.** Milestones (anniversaries, graduations, birthdays) can trigger very painful feelings even years and years later.

Contributions and gifts for the family...

After someone dies, folks will often want to express their sympathy by giving a gift of some sort. Some gifts offer comfort and support right away while others are meant to remember the loved one for years to come.

5

❖ **Flowers** A gift of flowers may be a beautiful tribute in some faiths and cultures, but in others, they may not be as well received at this particular time. If you are not sure, check with the family's place of worship, the funeral director, or a family friend.

❖ **Flowers from the garden** Some individuals or families may request flowers from home gardens instead of purchased arrangements.

❖ **Flowering perennial** Plant a perennial in the family's yard in memory of the loved one, of course with family approval.

❖ **Food** Baked goods or simple meals that require no preparation other than warming are a practical gift. In the Jewish faith, uncut fruit is appreciated. In the Buddhist religion, gifts of vegetarian food are welcomed.

❖ **Living trees** In the Jewish faith, a gift of a living tree is welcomed in lieu of flowers.

❖ **Park bench** Often families or groups will dedicate a bench in memory of an individual.

❖ **Books** These are donated to a library in memory of the individual, often with a special notation on the inside cover.

❖ **Mass cards** These cards are an offering of a mass (a full Catholic service including the celebration of Communion) said for the deceased. Mass cards can be obtained from any Catholic parish and sometimes from a funeral parlor.

❖ **Memorial contributions** (remembrances) Many individuals or families designate one or more organizations to receive donations in memory of the deceased.

❖ **Money donation** Money is a frequent sympathy gift in most traditions. The families may use the money to assist with living expenses, funeral expenses, or educational funds. In the Jewish faith, money donations featuring the number 18 or multiples of 18 are meaningful. In the Muslim tradition, money is given to help pay the family debts. In Japanese traditions, a money gift of crisp new or ironed bills (Koden) is given to help cover the cost of the funeral.

❖ **Novena** This is a Catholic ceremony that can include nine nights of prayer for the deceased.

❖ **Service project** Individuals or groups can offer time and service in the name of the deceased.

See also, "Remembering the deceased," page 115.

Ways to help right away...
Notifying others...

When someone dies, family members typically join together to notify others and to get assistance with the final arrangements. In other situations, the family may need a trusted, knowledgeable friend to quickly take the lead with some of the plans.

❖ **Notify clergy or religious leader.** Many families turn to the clergy for support at this time. Even more may request the help of a clergy member for performing the service/s.

❖ **Put together a list of people to notify.** This list would include immediate family, close family, and business colleagues.

❖ **Phone immediate family and friends.** Offer the use of a phone or long distance line (donated by an organization or an individual business) for family-related long distance phone calls.

❖ **E-mail out-of-town family and friends.** Important family members may use e-mail communication especially if they are traveling in or out of the country. An offer to loan a computer with Internet access may be helpful.

5

Assisting with burial or cremation decisions...

Following a death, the family will need to make some lasting decisions very quickly. As a friend, you may be asked to be there for support as they make decisions.

❖ **Clothes for the deceased** Clothing is always important to families when the body will be viewed.

❖ **Burial decisions** Casket, lining, cemetery, gravesite, grave marker, etc.

❖ **Cremation decisions** Crematorium, type of urn, location/s for spreading ashes, etc.

❖ **Items to be buried or cremated with the deceased person** Families may need support when they pick mementos to be buried with the body versus those to be kept by surviving relatives (jewelry, beloved keepsakes, pictures).

Gathering essential information and documents...

Most families do not have the vital documents in one easy-to-find place. So when someone dies, gathering important documents can be overwhelming. Again, the family may want help from a trusted and experienced friend.

❖ **Gather information needed for writing the obituary.** Most newspapers provide a form for basic information (age, place of birth, place of death, occupation, college degrees, memberships held, military service, outstanding work, lists of survivors, time and place of services).

❖ **Help family find important documents.** Essential information (organ donation requests, burial plans, wills, birth certificates, marriage licenses, social security numbers, military service papers) may be kept in file cabinets, safety deposit boxes, safes, or even in a shoebox under a bed.

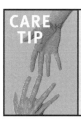

CARE TIP

Even if a family makes its own final arrangements, family members may still appreciate support from someone "just being there" and offering opinions only when asked.

Helping with immediate financial details...

Some folks have dealt with finances for a long time, while others have spent years having someone else do them. Ask if the survivor needs help with these types of details.

❖ **Access bank accounts.** A spouse may want to access bank accounts to withdraw funds for immediate use following a death. Offer to drive him or her to the bank.

❖ **Help the survivor track bills that need immediate attention.** Someone in grief may be too upset to pay attention to finances, especially if not experienced with paying the bills. But, bills still need to be paid. Consider having a trusted family member or friend offer to help sort through the bills.

❖ **Set up memorial funds.** People will want to know right away where to send monetary gifts in memory of the deceased. Memorial donations are commonly given to a church, hospital, disease-specific organization (American Cancer Society, American Heart Association, National Kidney Foundation), hospice, library, charity, school, service organization, or education fund.

5

Assisting family and friends who come into town...

During this upsetting time, someone who is good with people can lend a hand with visiting family and friends. This is a perfect opportunity for a calm and caring person to jump in and help.

❖ **Assist with transportation.** Close family and friends may be coming for services from out of town. Help may be needed to pick people up from the plane, bus, or train station and to take them to the home, funeral parlor, or funeral service.

❖ **Open your home for out-of-town family members to stay.** During a crisis, the family may not have room for everyone to stay. Offering a room is a very nice gesture.

❖ **Run errands for family members.** People who have rushed to get to a service may have forgotten important personal items (medications, personal care items). An offer to take someone to the store or to pick up necessities can be very helpful.

❖ **Provide childcare.** Family members who have come into town would appreciate an offer to baby-sit so they can grieve or attend services without worry.

Helping at the family's home...

After a death, family and friends may want to come by the home. Not all families, however, are ready for drop-in visitors and some may want their privacy. Regardless, many people may stop by or phone to offer support and condolences. Having someone spruce up the home, screen calls, and greet visitors can be a practical gift.

❖ **Organize people to sit with or spend the night with the person or family in grief.** Due to the initial shock and numbness of a death, some grieving family members may not want to be alone. Perhaps they would feel some comfort in having someone in the home to listen or to just be there.

❖ **Straighten up the house.** Most people are not always ready for company. Getting the house ready for out-of-town guests or drop-ins can be a godsend.

❖ **Answer door and greet visitors.** In some communities, neighbors and friends drop in as soon as they have heard the news of a death. It is helpful to have someone to answer the door to receive cards, flowers, gifts, and food items. With the family's approval, someone can also be present to answer any questions about the service or reception.

❖ **Screen and answer phone calls and messages.** After a death, the phone often "rings off the hook" with well-wishers as well as out-of-town family members needing information. Having someone at the phone will shield the family from having to repeat the same details over and over again and allow them to answer only essential phone calls.

❖ **Keep a record of visitors and calls.** Whether a formal guest book or sheets of notebook paper are used, a complete record of phone calls and visitors will be appreciated months down the road.

❖ **Keep a record of cards, flowers, food items, or gifts received.** The days immediately following a death are just a blur for many. Without some record of these kind gestures, they will likely be forgotten. While the family should not feel obligated to respond, a list of gifts brought by caring folks can be priceless.

❖ **Offer refreshments to visitors.** Some families will want to serve visitors who stop by the house, while other families will just wait for the reception. Ask the family for their preference.

5

❖ **Bring practical supplies to the family home.** Again, most people are not prepared to receive large numbers of folks. Check to be sure the family has basic paper products (toilet paper, tissues, paper plates).

Assisting with the service and reception...

People say a formal goodbye to a loved one in many different ways. Many have religious ceremonies, but some don't. Many have the service and the reception in the same place; some have the service in one place and the reception in another. Regardless, a final service and reception for a loved one is the most usual way that people say goodbye.

The grieving family will likely make most of the decisions for these gatherings as a way to begin to deal with the loss. For others, these decisions may be almost impossible to make. In either case, your help in carrying out the family wishes can be invaluable.

There is much to be done and many ways for people to help. Some folks are great with planning and setup while others are more comfortable working in the kitchen or playing with children. A close friend may be chosen to calmly help with some of the tough personal decisions. Helping with any of these details is a great way for people to show that they care.

Overall planning...

For some families, these arrangements will be easy to make. Others may have no idea what to do. In either case, many decisions will need to be addressed.

❖ **Determine the location for the service.** For some, the service will be held in a place of worship (church, synagogue, temple). Other services, whether religious or not, may be held elsewhere (mortuary, school, park, community center, hospital chapel, family home).

❖ **Choose a location for the reception.** If the family does not have a close connection with a religious community, they may not know where to hold a reception. Call to see what might be available (church, synagogue, temple, meeting hall, school, restaurant, community center, school, park, a friend's home) with a short notice.

❖ **Investigate service or reception charges.** Typically, there are charges for the facility, singers, ministers, and musicians. While close friends ~~~~~~~~ ~~~~te their talents, others may expect to be paid a fee. ~~~~~~~~ e someone else searching out this sensitive

~~~~~~~ t and supplies for the service and reception. y will have all the necessary equipment. In tificial or live plants, LCD or slide projectors, bles, chairs) will need to be rented·separately. e family before finalizing any costly rentals.

e reception. Arranging the room can include bles, chairs, plants, tents, or awnings, if out- g the room so that everyone can quickly get s as well as greet the family members.

❖ **Find people to direct traffic and parking where the service or the reception will be held.** Parking problems often delay people getting to the service or reception on time. When the attendance is expected to be high and the parking tight, this can be important!

❖ **Find someone to stay at the house to prevent burglary.** With obituary notices in the paper, the home becomes vulnerable to burglary. Find a trusted person, someone who is not a close friend or is willing to miss the service.

5

Tending to the family...

Just because a death has been expected doesn't mean that the family has prepared for what lies ahead. Many will appreciate a gentle, trusted friend or family member to help them through these personal details.

❖ **Find clothes for family members who will attend various services.** Due to lack of time or the need to travel, some family members may not have clothes they feel are appropriate. Consider loaning suit jackets, dresses, or accessories. Don't forget the children.

❖ **Assemble pictures or memorabilia of the deceased.** These displays reflecting the deceased's life are usually placed for viewing right before or after the service, at the home, or at the reception. While the family may want to choose their favorite pictures, they may want help setting up the display (photo table, picture wall, slideshow, audio-visual program).

❖ **Drive the family to the service.** If the mortuary does not provide transportation for the family, find someone who is trustworthy and will protect the family's privacy during this time when they are likely vulnerable. Be sure to clean the car first!

❖ **Find a private entrance to the service for family members.** Especially if family members are upset, they may need time before the service to collect their thoughts and emotions out of the public eye.

Planning the service...

Some families will have their religious leader assist them with all of these details. Others may need help in putting the pieces of the service together.

❖ **Contact close family members or friends to help usher.** In some cases, a family may be unable to handle this detail. Determine the number of ushers based upon the size of the service.

❖ **Assist the family in choosing pallbearers.** Avoid asking someone with heart or back problems to lift the casket. Instead, ask them to be honorary pallbearers.

❖ **Assist the family with the written program's design and copy.** Often, a written program will be given to those who attend the service. While some mortuaries have standard programs that can be used, some families will want to design their own.

❖ **Lead the service.** If the family does not have a religious leader to direct the service, someone will need to welcome guests, introduce speakers, offer a time for people to share their memories of the loved one, and finally, thank people for coming.

❖ **Help plan the order of the service.** While many families will have a clergy member or the mortuary assist them with the planning, families without professional assistance might appreciate help deciding what should happen from beginning to end. Libraries and websites may have useful information.

❖ **Arrange for singers, piano, or organ players.** A religious organization or the mortuary will likely have recommendations.

5

❖ **Plan for extra seating if needed.** Be sure someone is ready to add chairs if necessary.

❖ **Set up additional sound systems.** If seating will not be possible in the main area and people will need to be in adjacent rooms, set up a sound system.

❖ **Coordinate music for the service.** Some families like to play the deceased's favorite music as part of the service or reception. Be sure to test the music and sound system before the service.

❖ **Assist with eulogies.** Most families will want one or more folks to speak about their loved one. Family members may be too upset to ask people to speak and might need someone to help them.

❖ **Read tributes.** People who cannot come to the service sometimes write letters, telegrams, or poems that the family wants read in the service.

❖ **Make an audio or video recording of the service.** While this may seem unusual to some, many families choose to record the service as a cherished keepsake or for those who may not be able to attend. ***Get permission from the family first!***

❖ **Remind guests to turn off their cell phones or beepers.** Station someone at the door of the service to greet and remind folks.

❖ **Invite guests to the reception following the service.** Be sure to include the time, the name of the facility, address, map, and phone number for questions.

Answering questions about the service or rituals...

As a helper, you may be asked what type of burial and service has been planned. With direction from the family, you can dispel concerns and confusion with accurate information. If you are not familiar with a particular religious group's customs, you may want to find a religious leader, a family member, or a close friend to explain the individual's or family's traditions.

❖ **Describe what will happen in the service.** Both children and even adults may have questions about these plans. Especially younger people have little experience with rituals and services surrounding death. A simple description of the order of the service may calm fears.

❖ **Explain how folks can participate.** Just knowing that songs will be sung, prayers will be said, or that people will be invited to share their memories of the loved one will let folks know what to expect. Again, a simple explanation may help people feel more comfortable.

❖ **Answer any questions about the presence of the body or ashes.** For some people, a big concern is whether or not they will need to view the body. Explain how they can politely excuse themselves without being noticed if they don't want to.

Tending to the children...

Don't forget the young ones. When people are very upset, children can get lost in the shuffle.

❖ **Arrange for childcare during the service.** Find a trusted adult to watch children either on-site or close by. Be sure to let people know it is available and have someone there to escort the family to the nursery.

❖ **Answer the children's questions and concerns about the service.** Children will likely have a variety of questions about the service. For example, "What will occur?" "Will the body be present?" or "Will they be required to view the body?" As a helper, you may want to "check in" with kids you know.

5

Creating lasting memories...

Long after the service, a collection of sympathy cards, handwritten notes, stories, and cherished photos can be a comforting blanket during lonely times. The service and the reception can be the perfect opportunity to request and gather memories.

❖ **Provide guest books.** The family will want a record of those who attended. Have more than one available for larger services so that people can attend the service on time. It can be helpful to find a volunteer who will direct people to the guest book.

❖ **Provide a basket for cards.** Instead of mailing, often people will bring sympathy cards to the service. Be sure someone is assigned to get these cards to the family after the service.

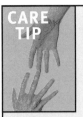

CARE TIP

When an adult child has died and has lived away from home, the parent may not know details about his or her friends and life. Even if a child still lives at home, the parents may not know about his or her impact on friends or teachers. Creating a "memory book" where people can enter special moments, stories, photos, or drawings about the deceased person can be comforting to the family.

❖ **Distribute and collect "memory cards."** Give those attending the service an opportunity to share a cherished memory or story of the deceased. As people sign the guest book, offer blank cards for them to write their thoughts. Provide a basket for the cards following the service. The cards can be left as they are, or nicely arranged in a "memory book."

❖ **Set up a memory book.** This can simply be a nice 3-ringed notebook with pretty sheets of paper inside. Have available quality paper, an assortment of pens, colored pencils, and markers. You may find that the reception is a more comfortable time for folks to write special memories of the deceased.

Sarah's story

Sarah lost her life when a car hit her as she was jogging down the road. The college held a memorial service for the staff and students. Sarah's elderly parents, who lived in another state, could not attend.

So, Sarah's closest friends decided to put together a memory book for her family. They included the program from the service and a collection of written memories, favorite moments, and funny stories written by the staff and students who knew her.

Sarah's parents treasured the book. It gave them a warm picture of Sarah's life away from home. The memory book also provided an opportunity for everyone at the school to get a bit of closure for themselves.

❖ **Take photos of the family.** Even though these are sad times, a service or reception will bring family members together from all over. For some, group and family photos taken now will not only bring comfort, but also mark an important family event. Only take photos with the permission of family members!

5

For information about planning food for a reception, see "Planning a fundraiser or a memorial reception," page 263.

Sharing flowers and food afterwards...

After the service and reception, there may be lots of extra flowers and uneaten food. What a shame to let it all go to waste! Even though family members might not be able to think about this themselves, they may appreciate knowing that someone did donate food or flowers in their loved one's name.

❖ **Donate flowers after the service.** Sometimes, a family cannot or will not want to take all of the flower arrangements home. So, ask the family if they would like any extra flower arrangements or plants delivered to special loved ones or places (helpful friends, nursing homes, retirement centers). Don't forget to take the gift cards off the donated arrangements. On each card, write a description of the arrangement for the family to look at later.

❖ **Collect and dry flowers from the service or gravesite.** Consider making fragrant sachets from the flowers lovingly given for the service. This can be a touching gift and a lasting memory, especially for folks who couldn't attend. Of course, ask first before taking some of the flowers. And then, ask the family for suggestions for the names of people who might appreciate this type of remembrance.

❖ **Donate any leftover food from the reception.** Often, there are lots of leftovers from any reception. Many places (shelters, youth centers, service organizations) routinely accept prepared food. Check to see if the family has other ideas. Always be sure to donate only unspoiled items.

Ways to help down the road...

When everyone returns to their routine, people who have lost a loved one may still need folks around them. Supporting them may mean carrying the load a bit while they are still numb, or it may mean walking along side them while they are facing a new life.

For some, a bit of help may tide them over until they are able to cope on their own. For others, an opportunity to learn everyday skills will help them be independent. For still others, a little bit of assistance on a continual basis may make the difference between someone staying at home or moving to an assisted-living facility. Be sensitive to what the surviving individual or family member needs and wants. *Ask.*

Remembering the deceased...

❖ **Mention the person's name and how they would have felt at a major milestone.** "Your mom would have loved to be here." "Your dad would be so proud of you." "Your grandmother would have loved this day."

❖ **Share wonderful stories about the person.** "Remember the time...." "I'll never forget when...." "I just loved her laugh when she...."

❖ **Make a quilt from the deceased's clothing.** Of course, this would be with permission only. This could include fabric from dresses, t-shirts with logos, suits, neckties, etc.

❖ **Make potpourri sachets from clothing or old lace handkerchiefs.** Some might really enjoy a pleasant fragrance every time they open the drawer.

❖ **Make new jewelry from the deceased's old beads.** Rejuvenate old jewelry by breaking up unusable strands and turning them into earrings, bracelets, or even tie tacks. *Do this with permission only!*

❖ **Return something that had been given to you by the deceased.** Especially when the survivor has very few keepsakes, a returned item may be very welcomed. For example, returning fishing gear to

5

a grandchild with the kind words, "Your grandpa would have loved for you to have this fishing pole," can be very special.

❖ **Organize a 1st year anniversary or annual fund-raising event.** Donate proceeds to the family or the deceased's favorite charity or interest. This should only be done with the family's knowledge.

Lynn's story

Ann was always known for knitting sweaters for newborn babies. She died when her daughter, Lynn, was very young. Years later, after Lynn married and was pregnant, a much older friend went to Lynn's baby shower. After the shower, she privately gave Lynn the sweater she had received from Ann years before.

❖ **Plant a flowering perennial, tree, or even a small garden in memory of the loved one.** This does not need to be done immediately following a death.

❖ **Make a cement stepping-stone with a loving tribute to the deceased.** This can be a lovely addition to a favorite garden.

❖ **Notify distant relatives and friends about the death.** There may be some people who still are unaware of the death even months down the road. A friend or relative may want to send out a letter, a copy of the program, or an obituary notice. They might even put together a notice with a picture of the individual and information about the last months/weeks of the person's life and final resting place.

See also, "Contributions and gifts to the family," page 99.

Remembering the living...

❖ **Allow the mourner to talk freely, to express feelings, and to cry.** Sometimes just "being there" without saying anything is a fabulous show of support.

❖ **Allow the mourner to follow his or her own grief timeline.** There are no set rules for how people will grieve or how long people will openly grieve. In fact, most people suffer major episodes of grief at key anniversaries or milestones during their entire lifetime.

❖ **Give an imaginary hug.** People who live far away and can only communicate by phone, letters, or e-mail can still support with loving words and thoughts. Tell the person on the other end of the phone, "I'm giving you a long-distance hug. Feel my arms wrapped tightly around you!"

❖ **Share your story if you have been through something similar.** Rather than dwelling on your own personal gloom and doom, talk about how you got through it. Be sure to give the person hope.

❖ **Give advice *only* if asked and *only* if you have been through something *very* similar.** For example, a grieving mother asked another who had also lost a child, "How did you survive?" The other mother was able to share from her own experience, "There will be days when you will feel the pain just as intensely as you are feeling it now, but you'll know you're getting better when there are more bearable days in between the horrible ones."

5

❖ **Bring two pieces of cake.** Or, bring two of anything to share, not just to leave behind. Very often the survivor is adjusting to loneliness. A bit of cake and conversation can mean a moment of warmth.

❖ **Welcome people back into the community.** Often people will not include a newly bereaved person in activities, thinking that she or he needs time alone. While some might need "alone time," others are desperate for ways to connect.

❖ **Acknowledge the siblings' loss, whether young or old.** Consider giving a special gift (video, CD, cozy blanket, framed photo or picture, book, stuffed animal).

❖ **Donate frequent flyer miles for airline tickets.** A time away might give the family members a chance to grieve away from the public eye.

❖ **Donate a private place for a family get-away.** Folks who own "time shares," a family condo, or a vacation home can help to provide a quiet respite.

❖ **Return pictures or videos of the deceased.** Sometimes folks have valuable pictures or videos that can mean so much to those left behind.

❖ **Plants or flowers** Either give flowers or plant some perennials outside in memory.

❖ **Fruit Basket** This can be a welcomed healthy alternative.

❖ **Audio books or CDs** Consider music or "talking books."

❖ **Notes and cards** A friendly note is always appreciated.

❖ **A phone call** Check to be sure someone is okay.

❖   **Tickets to a future event** Give them something to look forward to.

❖   **Meaningful passages, songs, or poems** These can bring comfort.

Making financial or legal changes...

Often, keeping financial and legal affairs in order has been one person's job. When that person dies, remaining family members will likely need to notify a variety of agencies and institutions (banks, credit unions, Social Security Administration, the deceased's stockbroker or financial advisor, and trade, fraternal, or military unions) about the death.

❖   **Funeral home or crematorium** In many circumstances, a death certificate will be required to make necessary changes. These are required for all legal and financial transactions. Obtain these from the funeral director or the Registrar of Vital Records in the area where the death occurred. The funeral director can usually help determine the number of copies needed and assist with obtaining them.

❖   **Post Office (U.S. Postal Service)** Notify the post office if there is a change of address or if mail needs to be forwarded.

❖   **Social Security Administration** When someone dies, Social Security Administration forms need to be completed to end the use of the deceased's Social Security number. To avoid any fraudulent use of the number, be sure to confirm that the Social Security number has officially been retired.

❖   **Landlord or mortgage company** In either case, arrangements will need to be made regarding payment, sale, or moving.

5

❖ **Utility companies** Again, these companies will need to be aware of the present situation and future arrangements.

❖ **Credit card companies** The bills will keep coming. Some people purchase special insurance coverage that will automatically cover all debts in case of a death. If not, consult with creditors and ask for more time to make payments.

❖ **All creditors** All debts, installment payments, and layaway purchases must be resolved.

❖ **Financial or tax advisor** Some people rely on an advisor. Be sure to notify the advisor about the death.

❖ **Motor Vehicle Department and auto insurance company** In some cases, the name on the automobile car title and insurance will need to be changed.

❖ **Life insurance company** Some folks will need help locating insurance information, changing names on policies, making arrangements for receiving benefits, etc. Monies from policies can be a lifesaver!

❖ **Lawyer** A death can bring many legal complications (wills, custody issues, lawsuits). Some folks will need help to obtain a good lawyer.

Mealtime...

Not everyone is familiar with the grocery store or the kitchen. If one person always did the cooking, the remaining spouse might welcome some help.

❖ **Coordinate people willing to bring food.** Even a home-cooked meal once a week might provide some company as well as a break from frozen food.

❖ **Assist or teach how to keep the refrigerator stocked, cleaned, and organized.** A refrigerator can be full with nothing to eat! Start with the basics, like checking for package dates and getting rid of old food.

❖ **Show how to shop for groceries.** When someone has never done this before, making a shopping list and picking out produce can be a challenge.

❖ **Teach how to prepare simple meals.** There are cookbooks that require just a few ingredients for a tasty dish! Pair up an easy-to-use cookbook with some free cooking lessons.

Household chores...

Again, some family members may never have learned how to do laundry or other basic household chores. Just a simple lesson may get them started.

❖ **Assist or teach how to do laundry.** Sorting whites from darks, choosing hot water or cold, delicate or regular...so many choices can overwhelm the novice. A few lessons can save someone from pink underwear!

❖ **Assist or teach how to clean house.** Dust keeps coming! A few basic hints and some standard cleaning products can save the day.

❖ **Bring in mail and papers.** A friendly neighbor who brings in the mail not only brings a bit of cheer, but can also check daily on an elderly person who has trouble getting around.

❖ **Set out and retrieve the trashcans.** Again, this may be hard for someone who has trouble getting around.

❖ **Water and mow the lawn.** A group of folks, perhaps a sport's team, a church group, or a community service organization can take turns.

5

Laura's story

When William, a high school social studies teacher, died of cancer, his wife, Laura, was overwhelmed by the responsibility of caring for her young son and maintaining her home. The school's track team promised to do all of the mowing for the summer until she could get on her feet. This not only helped with a time-consuming chore, but also gave little Billy time with some guys who would play ball with him once the lawn was cut.

❖ **Plant, water, and tend the garden.** For the person who lives for fresh vegetables, what a special gift!

❖ **Water and tend houseplants.** When someone is grieving, watering plants can be forgotten. Someone coming frequently to tend to the plants can be some company as well.

❖ **Care for pets or livestock.** Some animals require a lot of work. Offer to help out for a while or maybe just once a week for a breather.

❖ **Assist or teach how to make a simple household repair.** While most know how to change a light bulb, many folks need advice for fixing a drippy faucet or handling a sluggish drain.

Personal care...

When a caretaker (someone who provides daily physical care for a loved one) dies, the daily care must still go on. While more permanent arrangements are being made, caring friends and relatives can help out.

❖ **Coordinate people willing to provide personal care.** Providing personal care (bathing, dressing, feeding, hair care) for someone who is frail or disabled could be a godsend.

❖ **Assist or teach others how to perform home health care.** If you have some experience in health care, consider teaching family members how to prepare and give medication or administer treatments.

❖ **Check daily on the survivor.** Sometimes just a daily call or visit is all that is necessary.

❖ **Find professional home health care.** Even when people have the necessary financial resources, getting adequate home care can be a challenge.

Transportation...

It's important to get the living back on the road to independence. While giving folks a ride (to appointments, grocery store, or pharmacy) may be essential at first, consider teaching them the skills to be on their own.

❖ **Teach the survivor how to drive.** Even in this day and age, some folks have never driven. Offer to give driving lessons and help to get a license.

❖ **Teach them how to use the public transportation (bus, subway, train).** Reading a schedule, buying tokens, or buying a pass may seem simple to some, but terrifying for others who have never done it. Go along with them and teach each step along the way.

5

❖ **Fill the gas tank or show how to put gas in the car.** For some couples, this chore always fell to one person. If that person has died, the other may need someone to go with him or her to the gas station for a few times.

❖ **Help with or teach about routine car maintenance.** Without routine servicing (changing oil, checking tire pressure or brakes, winterizing), a car can quickly become unsafe to drive. Consider using a calendar to mark the dates for taking the car to the garage.

Teaching basic financial skills...

❖ **Use the bank.** This can include accessing bank accounts, getting loans, or even writing checks, etc. Though this is essential, it is often overwhelming for someone having to instantly take over.

❖ **Pay the bills.** Those monthly bills keep showing up no matter what. Come up with a simple tracking system so important bills are not forgotten.

❖ **Save and invest money.** This can be an overwhelming task for someone who has not paid attention to investments before.

Helping to get back into the job market...

When someone has died, the remaining spouse may need to get a job. Sometimes, she or he has not been part of the work world for a long time. A friend or relative may be able to assist with where to start and what to do.

❖ **Skill building** The individual may either need new formal training or just a bit of help to refresh skills prior to applying for work in his or her area of interest.

❖ **Resumé writing** People who have been out of the workplace for a while may not realize their potential or their marketable skills. A friend's perspective may be invaluable in creating a catchy resumé that can cinch a job.

❖ **References** You can't get a job without references! A friend can be a reference and may also suggest others who would be appropriate.

❖ **Job connections** Do you know someone who knows about a job? Doors open easier with a direct link.

5

┌───┐
│   │
│   **Note to helpers...**   │
│   To be sure all of your support is truly kind,   │
│   take a look at Chapter 6, "Caring without offending"   │
│   and Chapter 7, "What ***to*** say, what ***not*** to say."   │
│   │
└───┘

Now imagine...

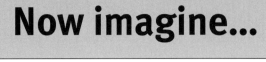

You have just found out that your coworker has died suddenly. After talking with the family and hearing that many family members will be arriving from out of town, the employees decide to provide meals for a week at the home. You volunteer to bring a spaghetti dinner for twelve on Wednesday.

Or imagine...

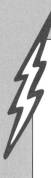

Your elderly aunt's son, your cousin, was killed in an auto accident. Now your aunt is alone and is faced with the many decisions regarding a funeral and reception. Up to now, the son has always been in close contact, visiting daily, running errands, taking her to doctor's appointments, and keeping her financial records organized.

You immediately go to her side and help her with all the funeral arrangements. After the services, you help her look at options for assistance at home. In addition, you plan to get together every week for dinner.

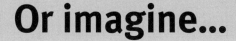

Or imagine...

Your neighbor and friend, an elementary school music teacher, has died after suffering from a difficult illness for several years. He leaves a wife and two teenaged boys. As a tribute to your friend, you decide to help coordinate the groups that have offered to help.

First, you contact the church where he belonged. His friends there offer to take care of the reception.

Next, you meet with the principal of his elementary school. Some of the teachers want to bring meals to the family. She will ask the school secretary to start a sign-up list and maintain a food donation calendar. She will also make reminder calls and answer questions.

Many classes of school children want to make cards for the family and you offer to deliver them to the home. Finally, you contact the president of the PTA, the parent-teacher association, because she has offered to organize a memorial scholarship fund. You make sure information about the fund is spread throughout the community.

5

PART II
Caring with true kindness...

CHAPTER SIX

Caring without offending...

In this chapter you'll find answers to...

- Why is it important for you to keep what you see and hear private?

- How can an illness or crisis change a patient and the family?

- How can you kindly keep from sharing details when asked?

- Why should you leave your own personal opinions at home?

6

Imagine...

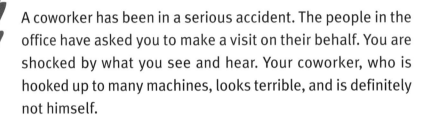

A coworker has been in a serious accident. The people in the office have asked you to make a visit on their behalf. You are shocked by what you see and hear. Your coworker, who is hooked up to many machines, looks terrible, and is definitely not himself.

When you return to the office, everyone wants an update. You don't know what to say. You are afraid that if you say too much, you will share more information than your coworker and his family want revealed.

Protecting privacy— keeping confidentiality...

The old saying, "Can you keep a secret?" is especially important when you have been helping during a health crisis. Confidentiality is critical!

Helpers will often see individuals and their families at a very vulnerable time. Once well, these people will need to face friends, neighbors, and coworkers. If graphic or private information has been shared, they will be embarrassed and uncomfortable, as will those around them.

In extreme situations, breeches in confidentiality may injure people's private lives and affect their ability to work. Everyone has a right to privacy!

The *patient* in crisis...

Remember that the ***patient*** might not seem like the person you've always known.

❖ **The patient may not be wearing his/her regular clothes.** Most likely the patient is in pajamas or in a hospital gown (with backside exposed). None of us would like to have a news bulletin go out about our bedridden fashion!

❖ **The patient may not be in the usual state of mind.** Someone who has experienced a major health crisis may seem very different (depressed, confused, going in and out of sleep or consciousness, heavily medicated, in shock, or experiencing memory loss from a concussion).

6

❖ **The patient may be in pain or reacting to pain medication.** Pain is not always controllable with medication and often when it is, side effects are likely. Confusion may result.

❖ **The patient may have major body changes.** An accident such as a fire, car accident, or bike accident can cause major changes to the body. Also, medications can take their toll, causing the face to get puffy or the body to bloat. Many diseases or medications can even cause changes in the color of the skin.

❖ **The patient may cry.** Sometimes patients are not able to control their emotions and may easily cry. Folks who have suffered the loss of a loved one, suffered a stroke, or have had any other severe condition often have times when they let down. They shouldn't be expected to "save face," be strong, or put on a good front.

❖ **The patient may lash out in anger.** Who wouldn't be angry about being sick or injured? Often people cannot contain their feelings and might even lash out at their dearest relatives or friends. Keep the incident to yourself and don't take it personally!

❖ **The patient may show a more intense side.** An illness or pain only tends to magnify a person's typical personality. The sad may get sadder and the angry may get angrier.

❖ **The patient may become frail.** An illness can rapidly weaken even the strongest. Multiple injuries, losses of blood, or severe treatments such as chemotherapy take a huge toll. People who are very proud and independent may now suddenly need help in the bathroom. They might also need help with walking, washing up, or getting dressed.

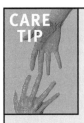

CARE TIP

If you are very upset by what you have heard or seen when helping in a health crisis, only share your concerns with someone you can trust (minister, counselor, close friend, relative) who will not tell others in the community. Think carefully... what would you want others to say about you and your family if you were the one in trouble?

The *family* in crisis...

Remember that the *family* might not seem like the family you've always known.

❖ **The family may be different than expected.** Family members living elsewhere often return home when someone is ill or injured. Their apparent lifestyle or physical appearance may take you by surprise. Remember, these family members and friends are vital people in the ill person's life and might be the key to a positive recovery. This is no time to be judgmental and no time to discount anyone.

❖ **The family may argue with each other.** Stress does not usually bring out the best in people. Old sibling rivalries and poor relationships often surface.

❖ **The family may not help as much as you might expect.** Some family members may be too stressed to help. Others may never have helped within the family and it becomes obvious now.

❖ **The family may not show up at all.** A health crisis may bring some families together, but often it does not. Some family members may stay away.

6

Jake's story

Jake has been in the same church choir with Nancy for years. When she recently suffered a severe stroke, Jake brought meals to the adult children who were taking turns staying with their mom while she was in the ICU (Intensive Care Unit).

One day, as Jake was setting out the food, the family members began arguing about the cause of their mom's stroke and blaming each other. Jake knew that Nancy would be mortified to know that he had heard her children bickering.

When he went to choir practice, everyone asked about Nancy. Even though Jake was very upset about what he had heard from Nancy's family, he just focused on Nancy's progress. He told them, "Her family is with her and she's getting a lot of physical therapy. Rehabilitation will take a long time."

Now's the time to keep a secret...

In a health crisis, you, as the helper, might see and hear private things.

❖ **You may overhear conversations about the individual in the hospital.** In a crisis, the helper may either overhear or be told personal details that may be private. Upset and vulnerable folks will often share information that they would not otherwise give out.

❖ **You may see, hear, or read medical information.** Even though health-care systems value confidentiality, personal health details may still slip out. For example, a visitor may notice a brochure or information packet left by the bedside that describes a particular medical condition. The patient may not want others to know that he or she has that condition. Discretion is so important.

❖ **You may find the home in disarray.** When a health crisis strikes, most people are taken by surprise and their home will likely not be ready for visitors. After a short while, even the best-kept place will look untidy. Most folks would be embarrassed to have others know about the home's condition.

Watch what you say!

What a helper says is powerful. Be careful what you say about the patient and the family. Your words can either help or hurt the individual and family for a long time to come.

When individuals come back to their routines after being sick, they want to be treated normally. They don't want people staring at them, thinking about how bad they looked when they were at their worst, or whispering about their chances for the future. People often treat someone who has gone through a bad experience differently.

The situation can only get worse if people have been...

❖   ...given a vivid description of how poorly the patient looked when he or she was really sick or injured.

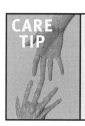

CARE TIP

The saying, "When in doubt, don't," applies when helping. It is better to err on the side of *not* sharing enough than telling too much!

6

❖   ...told how the individual or family members behaved during the crisis (crying, screaming, blaming).

❖   ...told that the individual will ultimately die from the illness.

Remember, no one (even a doctor) can accurately predict when someone will die, even though there may be a "guesstimate." People deserve and may need to maintain their routines while they can. They may need and want to carry on with their jobs, tend to their families, and get together with their friends. So, share only what is okay with the individual or family. Let them and let time tell the rest.

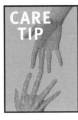

CARE TIP   As a helper, you ***do not*** have to tell "the whole truth and nothing but the truth." Let time tell the details. Preparing what to say ahead of time will make it easier to keep from sharing private information.

What can you say?

Both caring and just curious folks may ask many questions of the helper. If possible, ask the individual or family what they would like shared with others. Sometimes, time and the situation does not let this discussion happen. Keep your comments simple and leave out specifics. See if one of these examples works for you.

❖   "Things seem really tough for Brenda right now. Are you interested in helping in some way?"

❖   "It's really scary for Joe right now. We're all hoping for better news."

Cory's story

Cory, a young single guy, has his own small bicycle business. Sadly, he has been diagnosed with a fast-growing brain tumor that is usually difficult to treat. While the surgery was somewhat successful, the doctors have told Cory that his future is uncertain. Bill, a close friend, was with Cory when he got the shocking news.

In spite of everything, Cory desperately wants to return to his shop and continue his everyday routine as much as his illness will allow. Bill asks Cory what he should share with others about the illness.

When people ask, Bill says, "Well, you know that Cory had surgery. Now he's getting additional treatments and he's anxious to get back to his business. He hopes he'll see you in the shop soon."

❖ "Maria will be recovering for a long time. We'll all have to wait to see how things go. The family will need help with meals and errands. Can we call you?"

❖ "Jeff is going through a really difficult time. No one knows what will happen."

❖ "Rita is very ill. Right now she's not having visitors, but the family will appreciate a card."

❖ "Tony just had major surgery. We'll all know more in a few days."

6

❖   "Rosa was taken to the emergency room at the city hospital with chest pain. This all happened so suddenly. We should know more soon."

❖   "The family wants you to know that... (Put the general information that the individual or family has approved here.). They are so grateful for your prayers."

❖   "John will be happy you asked. After the accident, he had surgery. Now he's getting rehabilitation every day and he's looking forward to coming to work next month."

Leave your personal beliefs and feelings at home!

Whenever you come to help, you bring along your own set of beliefs and values. It's important to know what your beliefs are, so you can keep them in check and can be sensitive to the folks you are trying to help. Expressing your thoughts and feelings now, in the middle of a crisis, may only add to their sorrow and their guilt.

When helping, always put your own beliefs aside and focus on what the person or family needs. Sometimes, people are dealing with an illness that results from unhealthy choices. If you say, "You shouldn't have been... (smoking, drinking, eating fatty foods, using drugs)," you may be speaking the truth, but you are not showing compassion, which is what is really needed now.

These people will have enough troubles in their life. They will likely spend a lifetime second-guessing and torturing themselves with the question, "What would have happened if only we had quit... (smoking, drinking, using drugs, eating fatty foods)?"

John's story

Your friend Paula's spouse, John, caused a horrible car accident where several people were injured. The police believe that John was drunk. As you drive to the hospital, you are aware that you have strong feelings about people who drink and drive. You also believe that this accident could have been avoided.

But, still, you want to be a support to your friend. You know that she will need something to eat, so you stop off at her favorite fast-food restaurant and pick up a meal.

You find Paula sitting all alone in the ICU waiting room. She is distraught and crying. There has been no one there to support her. You just listen as she pours out her heart and her grief. In spite of your anger at John, you tell her you will be there for her, no matter what.

Always put yourself in the other person's shoes and imagine what you would be feeling if this situation had happened to you. By knowing who you are, what you believe, and by focusing on being compassionate, you will be more likely to truly help and not hurt.

Different strokes for different folks...

Some people have a strong sense of the rituals and traditions that bring them comfort during illness and tragedy. Others may not. Be sensitive and do not impose your own beliefs or traditions when people are struggling. Don't make assumptions about what will be helpful and comforting to someone else.

6

Joan's story

You believe that eating well and staying fit helps you stay healthy. Your coworker, Joan, who is very overweight and is a heavy smoker, has had a massive heart attack. She is in the ICU and is awaiting surgery.

Larry, Joan's husband, comes out of her room and into the ICU waiting room. When he sees you, he says, "I kept telling her to quit smoking," or "She had just started to lose weight." Instead of agreeing with him, and adding, "She should have quit a long time ago," you quietly say, "I am so sorry you are going through this."

Respect differences...

❖ **Ethnic group** Some ethnic groups speak different dialects and practice different customs depending on the region they come from. City folks may be very different from country folks. Those who live in the United States with its "Americanized" traditions may be very different from those who have recently immigrated to this country. However, during a time of crisis, some may fall back on the familiar traditions of their childhood.

❖ **Part of the country** Even within the U.S., there are major differences between those who live in the North or the South, the East or the West, or even the Midwest.

❖ **Religion** Just because people have grown up in a certain religion does not necessarily mean that they follow that religion now or follow all of its practices. On the other hand, just because people have veered away from their religious background in the past does not mean that they will not return to it during a crisis.

In addition, even within the same religion, some groups are more conservative while others are more liberal. Even some families who attend the same church, synagogue, temple, or mosque can vary in how closely they follow the traditional religious practices.

❖ **Age group** Each generation is shaped by its time and events.

❖ **Economic level** How much money someone has may dramatically affect the access to health care, the quality of insurance benefits, and personal choices surrounding a death.

❖ **Educational background** Education can affect a person's ability to provide self-care or a family's ability to care for the patient.

❖ **Family** Each family adds its own flavor to any set of beliefs.

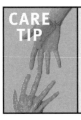
CARE TIP Care without offending! This is the time to *demonstrate* your love and concern. Be sensitive to individual differences and honor those beliefs.

6

Now imagine...

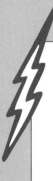

When you return to the office after having visited a coworker at the hospital, your officemates want an update. You don't want to describe the many scary details of what you have seen and heard. You know that if you were in your coworker's state, you would want people to respect your confidentiality.

So, instead, you just say, "He's going through a really difficult time right now. No one knows what will happen. Why don't we put together a meal for the family who is waiting at the bedside?"

Or imagine...

You are visiting your close friend's daughter in the hospital when the family gets the bad news that the daughter has a rare disease. The family members, of course, are very upset. The father doesn't like the doctor and wants a second opinion. Your friend, on the other hand, wants the treatments to begin right away. You witness their loud quarrel. As she walks you out to the car, your friend says, "I'm so embarrassed you saw all that."

You say to your friend, "I know this is a terrible time for you both. Please know that I won't share any of this with anyone. Still, I know that your friends will want to know how Sarah is. What would you like me to share?"

Or imagine this...

Mary, your very good friend, is dying. Everyone at the church wants to know what is going on, but Mary's family is reluctant to give out much information. Since so many people are calling the home, you ask if you can set up and maintain a phone hotline or an online social-networking page with updates and information about Mary. You assure the family that they would be able to approve all information before anything would be released. Then, people could call in or log on to the Internet for updates on Mary at any time without bothering the family. The family decides to let you give it a try.

So, you set up the phone hotline and a social-networking page and give a family-approved update about Mary. The family also asks you to add that they are grateful for people's kind thoughts and prayers.

6

What *to* say, what *not* to say...

In this chapter you'll find answers to...

- What are some easy steps for finding the right thing to say?

- How do you choose comforting words?

- Why are some often-heard phrases that are not so helpful?

Imagine...

You're at the grocery store and you see a neighbor whose child has been diagnosed with a terrible illness. You want to say something that shows you care, but you don't know what to say.

Easy steps for creating a comforting moment...

7

When someone is very ill or when someone has died, most people just want to say **something** helpful. However, it seems as though finding "the right thing to say" is the hardest task. Sometimes you have time to choose your words because you are planning to visit someone in the hospital or you know you are going to attend a funeral.

But, other times, you have no warning. You could be at the store or some event and run into someone who is suffering. Instantly, you need to come up with something helpful to say. Unfortunately, this is just when people are at a loss. It's not uncommon to freeze. Keep things simple.

For that on-the-spot moment, try these easy steps:

1. **Start with a warm greeting.** Smile and say, "Hi, Sarah. How are you doing?" (Be sure the tone of your voice shows you care.)

2. **Focus on the "hurting person" and acknowledge what he or she has been going through.** Try saying, "I was so sorry to hear you've been going through such a terrible time," "It seems so unfair," or "I was so sad to hear about your mom."

3. **Just listen if he or she needs to talk.** Someone who is hurting may need to talk without interruption and certainly without being told "everything will be okay."

4. **Leave with some positive words.** Try saying, "I'll sure be thinking about you," "Hang in there," or "Let's have coffee next week."

5. **Reach out with a warm gesture** (give a hug, touch his or her arm, shake hands).

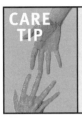

CARE TIP Ignoring someone who's going through a bad time is much worse than saying the wrong thing. If you are afraid you'll "choke up," just remember a hug or a soft touch can make up for any loss of words.

Comforting words...

Whether you have time to plan what you are going to say or are on "short notice," remember to focus on the hurting person, rather than ignoring the situation or talking about yourself. The following might be some helpful things to say.

Expressing concern...

These common expressions are often used. They are a kind way of saying that you have not forgotten him or her and that you are very concerned about how he or she is doing.

❖   "You're in my thoughts and prayers."

❖   "I'm thinking about you."

❖   "I haven't stopped thinking about you."

❖   "How are you getting along?"

❖   "How are things going?"

❖   "It must be so hard."

❖   "It's nice to see you. How are you doing?"

7

Showing compassion...

Although the next comments show your concern, they don't make the mistake of saying that you know exactly what the person in pain is feeling.

❖ "I hate that this is happening to you."

❖ "I'm sorry this is happening to you."

❖ "I'm so sorry you're going through this."

❖ "I'm so sad about this whole thing."

❖ "I can't imagine how you are feeling."

❖ "This hurts me to see this happening to you."

❖ "This seems so unfair."

❖ "This breaks my heart."

Charlie's story

Charlie has just been diagnosed with lung cancer after a lifetime of heavy smoking. He is devastated.

Mack, a friend from work, comes to visit. He listens as Charlie asks the question, "Why me?" Although Mack knows that Charlie's smoking habit likely caused this cancer, he comforts Charlie and says, "I'm so sorry you have to go through this."

Offering support...

Show you care with these comments. Some of these also mean that you are willing to listen or help in some way.

❖ "I'm praying for you."

❖ "I'm behind you all the way."

❖ "I care about you."

❖ "I wish you peace."

❖ "I'm here for you."

❖ "Would it be helpful for me to…?"

❖ "I'm here and I will be here when you need me."

❖ "I know you are going through a rough time. Just know I'd like to listen if you ever feel comfortable sharing."

Olivia's story

Shirley's husband died several years ago. When her friend, Olivia, lost her husband, she remembered how hard it was to do all of the necessary paperwork.

The week after the service, she said to Olivia, "After Harvey died, I was overwhelmed by all of the paperwork I had to do. Would it be helpful for me to come by next Tuesday afternoon and help you start to sort it all out? And then, if you want, we can set up a time each week to work on it until it is all done. I'll bring a dessert for us to share, too."

7

Providing encouragement...

These are perfect if you know the person well or if you have seen positive changes over time.

❖ "It's so nice to…(see you smile, hear you laugh, see you back at work, see you walking your dog again)."

❖ "I admire your…(courage, strength, patience)."

❖ "It's so good to see that you are getting along."

❖ "It seems like you're doing a good job putting one foot in front of the other."

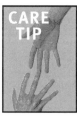

CARE TIP When you say something in an effort to comfort someone in grief, don't always expect a reply. Survivors may be in too much pain or not have the energy to respond.

Providing encouragement when someone has died...

❖ "I will always remember the time when Sam…(Use something positive or funny here — ***not something negative***.)."

❖ "Laurie…(was so important to me, taught me important lessons, always made me laugh)."

❖ "I believe that Bill is still with us."

❖ "I will never forget Anne."

❖ "When my child died, I got through it by…"

❖   "There will be days that will be just as intense as the pain you're feeling now, but you'll know you're getting better when there are more good days in between the bad ones." ***Only someone who has "been there" can say something like this***.

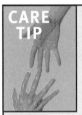 **CARE TIP**   Sometimes, people who are hurting are just trying to put one foot in front of the other. They still have to go to work or run errands without falling apart. They may dread having to face people and to respond to their words of comfort ***in public***.

If you think this is the case, don't ignore the person when you see him or her. Instead, try just giving a nod or a warm touch on the arm as you walk by. And then, show you care by calling, sending an encouraging note or e-mail, or a gift ***to the home***.

Not so helpful words...

When we see someone suffering or grieving, we want to say something kind and supportive. Our intentions are ***always good***, but the words we choose may not be. Often, we are uncomfortable and afraid we will say the wrong thing. Then, our words can spill out in nervous talk. We may quickly rely on pat phrases we have heard before. While familiar, these commonly heard words might not give the kind and sensitive support we would hope.

Often heard, but often hurtful words...

Not knowing what to say, people often repeat "the old standbys," or things they have heard others say in similar situations. These comments are often hurtful:

7

❖ **"I know how you feel."** Unless you have had a very similar personal experience, you can't begin to understand how someone feels.

❖ **"God only gives you what you can bear."** This is ***not*** comforting for people who are suffering. They will wish that God had less faith in their endurance.

❖ **"If you had only...(gone to the doctor, taken care of yourself, heeded the warning signs), this would not have happened."** This is no time to fill the person with regrets. Undoubtedly, she or he has them already.

❖ **"That's what happens when you... (smoke, drink, don't wear seatbelts)."** Even though a person's behavior or choices likely contributed to his or her illness, comments such as these are cruel and judgmental.

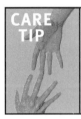

| CARE TIP | If you have been through something similar, give the person hope by talking about how you got through it. Be careful not to fill him or her with your own horror stories, your fears, and your gloom and doom. Focus on being helpful! |

❖ **"You shouldn't feel that way."** There is no rule that says how someone should feel.

❖ **"Aren't you feeling better yet?"** This gives the message that you have a timeline or expectation for the person's sadness.

❖ **"When are you going to get back to being the person I once knew?"** This implies that you cannot accept his or her present state. The person has probably been profoundly changed and may not ever be the same.

Paula's story

Paula and Jan have been fast friends since their teenagers were babies. But, ever since Paula's daughter was tragically burned on the face two years ago, the two have not spent much time together.

Jan aches as she remembers their long chats over coffee and laughing at their kids' antics. Because of her own sadness, she wishes she could ask Paula, "When are you going to get back to being the person I once knew?" Given what's happened, however, Jan knows that things between them may never "get back to normal."

So, instead, Jan simply says, "I miss you. I miss our weekly chats and all the laughs we used to have."

❖ **"Aren't you over it yet?"** Major accidents, illnesses, and grief can affect an individual for a lifetime.

❖ **"It's time to move on."** Maybe the person is unable to move on due to the depression that typically follows a major trauma or illness.

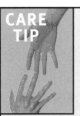
CARE TIP

Sometimes a person who has been "hit by life" will really struggle to "move on." If you are so concerned that someone very close to you is immobilized by grief (not eating, not sleeping, not bathing, not going to work, isolating from others), you may want to contact the person's family doctor. In addition, you may want to find someone who has "been in their shoes," or you may try to locate a welcoming support group.

❖ **"I don't know how you go on."** While this is likely meant to be a comment of admiration about the person's endurance and courage, this is not an encouraging comment. It may sound like anyone in this situation shouldn't go on.

❖ **"I'm glad it's you and not me."** While this might be what most people would think at hearing of a tragedy, why would anyone say this?

❖ **"You have the strength to go through this. I wouldn't be able to do it."** Again, anyone hearing this might think, "If being strong is why this happened, then let me please be weak!"

❖ **"You look so...(tired, weak, pale)."** Even though this may be true, this type of statement can only alarm the individual and cause him or her to dwell even more on the illness.

❖ **"You must be so...(miserable, afraid, angry)."** Again, though this may be true, this type of statement forces feelings on someone else.

❖ **"This will be over soon."** This statement could be misinterpreted many ways. For example, does it mean that the patient will die soon? Does it mean that the person will get better? How could anyone know?

❖ **"It'll be okay."** How would anyone know what will be okay?

❖ **"You can beat this."** How would anyone know that this is true? Also, some people with a long-term illness prefer to think in terms of "living with the illness" rather than "beating the illness."

7

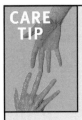

CARE TIP Remember, any comment can be misinterpreted. Be patient if someone seems to have taken your words in a way you did not intend. Stress, lack of sleep, medication, and the pain of terrible circumstances often affect how people hear things.

If you do say something that you think has caused pain, intentionally or unintentionally, clear up the misunderstanding. Don't ignore the problem. For example, you could go back to the person and say, "I think I may have said something that hurt you, and I'm so sorry if it did. What I meant was..."

Words *not* to say when someone has died...

Even though the following comments carry a bit of truth, someone whose heart has been broken does not need to hear them. Such a comment sounds like you don't begin to recognize his or her raw pain or loss.

❖ **"You can always have another baby (husband, wife, friend)."** You can't replace a person just like getting a new loaf of bread at the store.

❖ **"At least you had him for fifteen years."** The person in grief never feels it is enough years.

❖ **"At least he isn't suffering."** While this comment may be true, the mourner will have mixed feelings. He or she may be relieved that the suffering is over, but at the same time be devastated that the loved one is gone.

7

Words that can be taken the wrong way...

Depending on a person's situation or religious beliefs, these comments can bring great comfort or be very upsetting. Be sure that you use these comments **only** when you are sure they will bring comfort.

❖ **"There's a reason for this to have happened."** Even though people may believe that everything happens for a divine reason, saying so might bring little or no comfort at this moment. People in pain may find this comment upsetting and offensive because they don't believe that they have been individually targeted for any reason. This comment likely comforts the speaker more than the ill or injured person.

❖ **"Keep up the good fight."** Someone might need these words of encouragement to face a tough treatment. On the other hand, if the person's condition is spiraling downward, "keeping up the good fight" may no longer be an option. These words may sound as though the person is not trying hard enough or long enough. Then, a comment like this can just bring guilt.

❖ **"He's in a better place."** Many faiths teach that this is true. So, for some, this comment can be very reassuring. However, remember, the person grieving naturally misses the loved one and would probably prefer him or her to be in **this** place.

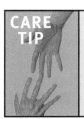

CARE TIP

Use these phrases cautiously as they can be taken the wrong way! Only use them if the hurting individual or family does first. Let them take the lead.

Now imagine...

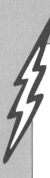

Steve runs into Jerry at the gas station as he is getting his morning cup of coffee before work. Steve has heard that Jerry's son, Billy, was just diagnosed with a brain tumor. Steve really knows very little about the situation, but feels like he ought to say something. Steve says, "Oh, man, I just heard about Billy. How's it going?"

Looking very distressed, Jerry shares some of the details with Steve while they are standing in line to pay for the coffee. When Steve gets to the front of the line, he pays for two cups of coffee, hands one to Jerry and tells him, "Cathy and I will sure be thinking of you. You will be in our prayers every night."

Or imagine...

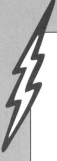

A month later, Steve sees Jerry at the gas station again. Now, Billy has had several rounds of radiation, surgery, and chemotherapy. Jerry now looks exhausted. Steve is at a loss for words as he tries to imagine the same thing happening to his son.

Steve again asks Jerry how he's doing. Jerry replies, "Not good. Billy is so sick, and we practically live at the hospital.

We're not sure what's going to happen." Steve shakes his head and says to Jerry, "I'm so sorry you're going through this." On the way home, Steve swings by Jerry's house, sees that the lawn is overgrown, and decides to bring his mower over after dinner to take care of it.

Or imagine this...

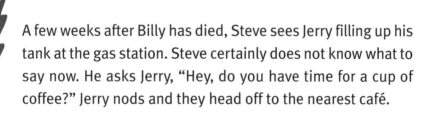

A few weeks after Billy has died, Steve sees Jerry filling up his tank at the gas station. Steve certainly does not know what to say now. He asks Jerry, "Hey, do you have time for a cup of coffee?" Jerry nods and they head off to the nearest café.

After rehashing last night's baseball game, the conversation came around to Billy and how he loved baseball. They both were able to laugh as Steve said. "Hey, remember the time when Billy totally ripped his uniform when he slid into home plate and then refused to get up?"

PART III
Everyday gestures...

CHAPTER EIGHT

Feeding the body and soul...

In this chapter you'll find answers to...

8

- When is a good time to bring food as a gift?

- What are some quick and convenient snack ideas?

- What are the steps for providing a complete meal?

- What are some types of tasty meals?

Imagine...

A friend's daughter has received a terrible diagnosis and will be in the hospital for major surgery and treatments. Family members arrive to be at the bedside. You know they will not want to leave the hospital and will need to have something to eat. You want to help by bringing some food, but don't know where to start.

Food for the family— a gift beyond nutrition...

A gift of a snack or a meal is much more important than the nutrition it brings. It sends along a kind wish that lingers with every bite, giving warmth and strength, even if the helper is not there.

When a crisis occurs, family members and very close friends can be overwhelmed. They will likely have no thought for their own needs and will find themselves running on adrenaline just to deal with their drastic circumstances. They may be reluctant to leave the bedside or waiting area to eat, hoping to get a chance to see their loved one or to talk with a health-care professional. We must nurture struggling families with snacks or meals as they cope with a health crisis.

When a health condition lasts over a long period of time, a random meal can be sweet relief for exhausted caregivers. Even better, a scheduled weekly or monthly meal is something for them to look forward to. In short, whether it's an immediate crisis or a chronic situation, people need help. Rough times such as these provide a great opportunity to be there to make a difference.

8

Times when food can be helpful...

❖ **Immediate hospital emergency** (heart attack, stroke, accident, pneumonia, birth with complications, mental-illness episode). During an emergency, people lose all sense of time. It either zooms by or passes so slowly, it's agonizing, especially if waiting for information. Family members or close friends may not realize how long it has been since they have had anything to eat or drink. They need to be encouraged to eat well and to drink plenty of fluids during a time of crisis so they can hang on.

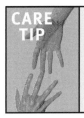

CARE TIP Don't forget any children or elderly folks at home who cannot come to the hospital. They may be sitting at home without the usual family cook.

❖ **Planned hospital stay** (for scheduled surgery, diagnostic tests, ongoing treatments) Even though planned, relatives probably have passed anxious hours in the waiting room or at the bedside without anything to eat or drink. Help take the pressure off by providing food, not only for those in the hospital, but also for those at home.

❖ **At-home recovery** (from trauma, surgery, illness, newborn with complications returning home) With the stress of someone being sick and the need to set up care at home (getting supplies, filling prescriptions, arranging the home to make care possible), figuring out the next meal may seem overwhelming. If you are helping or visiting, bring along some healthy beverages and snacks. If the pantry is empty, you can make a quick run to the store, quickly prepare a simple meal, or have something delivered.

❖ **Sporadic bouts with a chronic illness** (emphysema, cystic fibrosis, severe asthma, muscular dystrophy, cancer relapse) Even though another attack of a chronic illness may be expected, it still can wear out a family. Some helpers might be distressed when they're faced with the

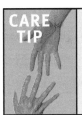

CARE TIP Respect privacy and wishes. Sometimes people want to be alone with their troubles, and other times people want company. For some people, cooking is a burden, but for others, the routine of cooking might be comforting in the midst of a crisis. *Ask first.*

grim reality that sometimes "things just don't get better." Regardless, people are struggling. Jump in to help.

❖ **Worsening complications of aging** (deteriorating joints, vision problems, confusion, poor appetite, isolation) Most of us know elderly people who are trying to cope with the day-to-day problems of aging. Many of the elderly no longer have folks who can support them. Their friends may no longer drive. Their family may live far away. A bit of help, a meal now and then, will not only provide them with good nutrition, but also will give them comfort and keep them connected.

❖ **Anxious time before death** When someone is dying, there is really very little anyone can do to relieve the pain. However, people can provide some comfort by bringing gifts of food. Again, death is a hard subject for all of us, but reaching out at this time is so helpful.

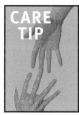

CARE TIP	Often a health crisis or a death brings extended family members together from far away. Imagine how comforting it could be to gather together for a home-cooked or catered meal in a private setting before everyone has to travel back home.

❖ **Immediate period after a death** Following a death, family members should be able to grieve and make final plans. They shouldn't have to worry about shopping or preparing food for friends and extended family coming into town. Providing them with meals gives them the needed time.

❖ **Blood drive** A bit of food and fruit juice is essential immediately after giving blood. If help is needed to cover the costs of lingering medical expenses, consider adding a fundraiser to the blood drive by having a bake sale at the same time. ***Of course, ask the family first!*** See "Planning a fundraiser or a memorial reception," page 263 for more information.

❖ **Fundraisers** Whether raising money for a transplant, trying to cover hospital expenses, or remembering a loved one, people are gathering to make a difference. Sometimes food is "the fundraiser" (spaghetti dinner, pancake breakfast) or is just an added attraction (popcorn at a carnival). Regardless, food always adds a festive note. See "Planning a fundraiser or a memorial reception," page 263 for more information.

❖ **Reception after a death** Bringing and serving food is a way to show support to the family and to honor the one who has died. See "Planning a fundraiser or a memorial reception," page 263 for more information.

❖ **Traveling care package** Often families need to travel a distance to visit someone sick or after someone has died. They face a plane trip or an anxious road trip without a meal. A quickly assembled assortment of snacks or an on-the-go meal could brighten dark moments.

❖ **Sensitive circumstances** (suicide, major mental illness, dementia, AIDS) Some individuals and families may be embarrassed about a crisis, not knowing how the news will be received. Now more than ever, reaching out and giving a gift of a meal can smooth over a rough time and let them know "you're there" for them.

Bringing snacks—food on the run...

Distraught family members may not be able to face the thought of a full meal. They may be waiting for news about their loved one and unwilling to leave the waiting room. A "care package" of individually-wrapped snacks that are easy-to-eat and easy-to-store can be invaluable.

When there's an emergency, supportive friends may only have a few minutes to gather items that might be needed in the hospital. The list below, "Convenient snack ideas," offers some simple and quick ideas. No need to bring the entire list of food items. Just grab a couple of things from the kitchen or make a quick trip to the store. Items that are individually packaged and don't require refrigeration or freezing tend to be the best as they are easy to store.

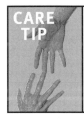

CARE TIP

Remember to include both nutritious food to keep them healthy, as well as a bit of "junk food" to provide comfort.

8

Convenient snack ideas...

❖ Individually-sized drinks (Consider juices or flavored waters for better nutrition.)

❖ Instant coffees

❖ Freshly brewed coffee (from home or a local coffee house)

❖ Teas

❖ Hot chocolate

❖ Fresh fruit

❖ Fresh vegetables

❖ Dried fruit (cranberries, raisins, assortments)

❖ Crackers

- ❖ Cheeses

- ❖ Pretzels and mustard

- ❖ Doughnuts

- ❖ Bagels

- ❖ Microwaveable popcorn packages (Caution: Some hospitals restrict microwaveable popcorn to certain locations as it can set off fire alarms if not well-attended during cooking.)

- ❖ Single-serving packages (tuna, chicken, seafood salad)

- ❖ Single-serving microwaveable soups or foods (the just-add-water variety or those that are ready-to-go)

- ❖ Yogurt (requires refrigeration)

- ❖ Hard-boiled eggs (require refrigeration)

- ❖ Individually-packaged puddings

- ❖ Fruit cups

- ❖ Fruit leathers or roll-ups

- ❖ Nuts

- ❖ Gorp (a homemade mixture of dried fruit, nuts, chocolate candies)

- ❖ Candy

❖ Gum

❖ Cookies (Don't forget graham or animal crackers!)

❖ Chips (individually packaged or in hard containers to avoid breakage and storage problems)

Snacks can be brought by the handful or cheerfully packaged in small baskets or decorated shoeboxes. Kids can help here!

8

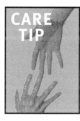

CARE TIP

In some hospitals, juice, tea, or coffee are free and available in the waiting rooms. Check first.

Bringing meals—a time for a break...

It's hard to live on snacks when you are used to three meals a day. Unfortunately, hospital cafeterias and coffee shops are often closed during the evening or wee hours and families are left with only vending-machine-type food.

On the other hand, when a sick family member is being cared for at home, caretakers may have little time or energy to think up the next meal. So, it is helpful for caring folks to supply some type of meal, even if it isn't home-cooked.

A meal can provide an important moment of respite from the stressful situation or trauma. When family members gather for a meal, they get a small window of time to relax and talk. The gift of a meal not only nourishes the body, but also the mind and reminds the caretakers that they are not alone.

Steps for making a complete meal...

While many people are familiar with cooking for their own families or themselves, they may not have ever prepared, packaged, or delivered a meal for someone who is sick or for a patient's loved ones. To be successful and to bring a meal that is gratefully received, there are several steps to consider.

Getting the facts first!

A meal that works for the whole family (takes into account food preferences, allergies, special diets) will hit the spot!

❖ **Ask the family about food preferences.** Bring meals that are comforting and not unusual to the family. Stay away from exotic and untried recipes and be sure to consider the family's cultural or ethnic habits.

❖ **Ask the family about special diet needs or food restrictions.** Many people are on a special diet for health reasons. If you are unsure how to prepare food for a particular diet, you may find helpful recipes in the library, bookstores, or on the Internet.

❖ **Ask the family about food allergies.** Some people have significant food allergies that could cause real distress in an already difficult situation. List all ingredients on the container if you have any doubts.

❖ **Find out the number of servings to provide.** Don't forget to include any extended family members who may be in from out of town. Also, consider packaging extra servings for the family's freezer if they have room.

❖ **Avoid foods with strong odors.** Be considerate of other patients and families on the unit! While foods with strong odors might smell wonderful to folks who are used to them, they can be very disturbing to others who are sick, injured, or distressed.

❖ **Choose food carefully for the elderly and the very young.** Some (not all) elderly folks prefer easy-to-chew and easy-to-digest foods. Also, many children are more likely to eat foods that are familiar, simple, and not spicy.

8

❖ **Designate a meal coordinator.** If many folks want to take turns bringing meals, it's great to have someone coordinate the schedule. The coordinator should be prepared to also answer questions about the family's food preferences and how to expertly prepare, package, and deliver the meal. This way, the family won't have to answer questions repeatedly.

Putting together the menu...

A complete meal typically includes many of the parts listed below.

❖ **Main dish** Check the family's food preferences before starting. Be sure you know if they are vegetarians or allergic to any types of foods.

❖ **Vegetables** These can be raw, steamed, or cooked into a favorite side dish.

❖ **Fruit** Fruit comes packaged by Mother Nature! If not eaten with the meal, a piece of fruit can be saved for later.

❖ **Salads** After eating vending-machine meals, salads (lettuce, bean, fruit, gelatin) can be a refreshing alternative. With a green salad, don't forget to include a small jar of homemade or commercial salad dressing.

- ❖ **Bread** Rolls and muffins are great. Butter and jam in individual packaging or small, disposable containers would be nice, too.

- ❖ **Dessert** Some meals just beg for a dessert! Cookies, brownies, and other finger foods are easy to handle.

- ❖ **Beverages** Hospitals offer limited choices for drinks, usually water, soda/pop, black tea, or coffee. Consider bringing in herbal teas (bags or bottled), flavored instant coffee, individually-packaged juices, seltzers, or bottled water.

Complete Meal Shortcuts

When time is short, you still may want to provide a complete meal with a homemade look. For example, you may only have time to prepare just a dessert or your favorite main dish. Or, you may not want to cook at all.

Consider some of these shortcuts:

Main dish
- ☐ Store-prepared from your grocery store or deli
- ☐ Frozen (from the grocery store, deli, or your own freezer)
- ☐ Take out (ethnic food, pizza, sandwiches, home-style foods)

Vegetables
- ☐ Store-prepared from your grocery store or deli
- ☐ Frozen (from the grocery store, deli, or your own freezer)

Fruit

☐ Pre-cut and packaged at the grocery store or deli

Salad

☐ Prepared and packaged at the grocery store or deli
☐ To make a leafy green salad look homemade, buy a package of lettuce and add toppings (tomatoes, cucumbers, carrots, croutons)

Bread

☐ Frozen or refrigerated dough, ready-to-bake
☐ Store-bought (deli, bakery, grocery store)

Dessert

☐ Ready-to-bake mixes (cake, brownies, cookies)
☐ Frozen (pies, cakes, bars, ice cream)
☐ Pre-packaged (cookies, cakes, candy, brownies)
☐ Store-made (deli, bakery, grocery store)

Beverages

☐ Teas
☐ Coffees
☐ Juices
☐ Powdered mixes
☐ Carbonated drinks

8

Preparing the meal...

This part is important! When people are dealing with a crisis, the last thing they need is to get sick. So, be sure you follow the basics rules of cleanliness and then keep the food at the right temperatures.

❖ **Don't prepare food if you are sick or getting sick.** Even if you have signed up to prepare dinner for the day, cancel or switch with someone else so that you don't bring your illness to the family you are trying to help.

❖ **Wash your hands.** Scrub for ten to fifteen seconds before you rinse your hands. Anytime you touch raw meat, you will need to wash your hands again before touching other food.

❖ **Clean the counters, cutting boards, and utensils carefully before beginning.** Then, be sure to rewash everything after working with raw meat.

❖ **Keep the food at a safe temperature.** Bacteria will grow quickly at lukewarm temperatures. So, hot foods need to be kept hot or quickly refrigerated if not served immediately. Cold foods also need to be refrigerated immediately and not just left out on a counter.

❖ **Clean all fresh fruits and vegetables.** Thoroughly wash and rinse all fruits and vegetables.

❖ **Cut food into individual portions.** For example, divide up grapes into small clumps, and slice cheeses, carrots, and celery. While casseroles can be spooned out, you may want to pre-cut hams, chickens, or roasts to make it easy for people to serve themselves.

Packaging the meal...

Packaging a meal is like planning a picnic. Keep it simple!

❖ **Bring only enough food for a meal or two.** Hospitals often have very limited, if any, refrigerator space.

❖ **Put all food in disposable containers.** The family should not have to worry about breaking dishes or returning them. If well-meaning people do bring meals in non-disposable baking/serving dishes, someone should be designated to clean, sort, and return any containers left at the home or hospital.

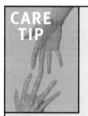

CARE TIP

People willing to donate food items may not have disposable containers for storing and transporting food. Ask others to save their empty containers (from individually-frozen entrees, whipped topping, butter, margarine, yogurt). This is a great project for churches, corporations, or service organizations that provide meals to individuals and families on a frequent basis.

❖ **Use ovenproof and microwaveable disposable containers for baking main dishes or casseroles.** These can be baked in the oven at home and then reheated at the home or hospital.

❖ **Store raw fruits and vegetables in resealable clear bags or empty plastic containers.** Prepared salads, raw vegetables, or washed fruit travel well in resealable bags or used plastic containers (from whipped topping, butter, margarine, yogurt products).

❖ **Put sauces or liquids in separate containers.** Wait to add any juice, drippings, or sauces to meat or salad until after delivery. Sloppy foods don't travel well!

❖ **Label and date all food containers.** Include not only the name of the dish, ingredients, and the date it was prepared, but also the warming or cooking instructions.

❖ **List significant ingredients.** Alert allergic people to contents (nuts, eggs, fish, shellfish).

❖ **Package foods carefully if freezing for later.** Freezer burn makes food inedible! Wrap the food tightly. Also, remember to label, date, and include reheating instructions for all packages bound for the freezer.

❖ **Bring beverages in disposable containers.** Consider purchasing juices or beverage drinks packed individually, in half-gallon cardboard containers, or in plastic two-liter bottles that can be simply thrown away when empty. Of course, individually-packaged herbal teas (bags or bottled), flavored instant coffee, juices, bottled water, or seltzers are always an easy solution.

❖ **Store food in a cooler.** If you're unsure if there will be refrigerator space and the food could sit out before being eaten, bring a new disposable cooler or a *very clean* one from home. This will be handy for leftovers as well. Disposable coolers are available in many grocery and general stores.

❖ **Include the necessary supplies.** A portable meal is so much more convenient if you bring serving, storing, and cleaning supplies.

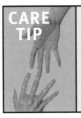

CARE TIP

Hospitals may provide refrigerator space for family use. In addition, some may provide coffee, tea, cocoa, etc. Check with the hospital personnel for rules about the available refrigerator space, foods, ice, and paper supplies.

Checklist of Handy Supplies to Bring With the Meal

☐ Disposable or easy-to-wipe table covering (perfect for laying out the food items)
☐ Disposable paper plates
☐ Disposable cups
☐ Disposable plasticware (forks, spoons, knives)
☐ Sharper kitchen knife for fruit and cheeses
☐ Paper napkins
☐ Paper towels for spills or clean up
☐ Individually-packaged sanitizing hand wipes
☐ Extra resealable bags for leftover food items
☐ Extra plastic wrap or foil to cover leftovers
☐ Plastic trash bags
☐ Soapy washcloth in resealable bag (for wiping off table covering, jars, etc.)
☐ Ice or re-freezable blue ice
☐ Small ice chest (Buy a new *small* Styrofoam chest or bring a used one that has been cleaned inside and out to store the leftovers.)
☐ Permanent marking pen for labeling leftovers

❖ **Make up a card to accompany the meal.** List the names of folks who provided the nourishing meal and send along warm wishes.

Delivering the meal...

Whether you are providing a home-cooked meal or a build-your-own sandwich/salad bar, delivery can be quite the trick! Getting it there all in one piece is crucial. Drive carefully. People are hungrily waiting!

8

❖ **Package meals so hot foods stay warm and cold foods stay cold.** To keep fresh-out-of-the-oven food warm, wrap the baking dishes in towels and fit them snuggly in a box. Put cold foods straight from the refrigerator to a cooler with ice or cold packs.

❖ **Put down a protective layer in your car.** Fresh newspaper or an old *clean* plastic tablecloth or tarp will work great. This will not only protect your car from spills, but also keep the food free from animal hair and dirt if you haven't had a chance to clean your car.

❖ **Prevent spilling food in your car.** You don't want your favorite creation to end up splattered all over the car. Put the hot dish, pie, or other spillable food items inside a cardboard box. If the item does not fit inside the box tightly, you can then roll up newspaper along the sides to stabilize the dish. The box will not only keep the casserole from spilling into the car, but will help keep it warm and make the dish easier to carry.

❖ **Wedge everything tightly on the car floor or in the trunk.** Use anything like rolled-up blankets, blocks of wood, or other boxes to keep the meal steady as you drive. You don't want to destroy all your hard work when you turn corners or need to stop quickly.

❖ **Bring hot pads and wet cloths.** These will be handy to clean up any spills that may still occur.

Serving the meal...

Sometimes a situation is so new or so stressful that the family members need to be gently reminded to eat and would benefit from being served. On the other hand, if the situation has been ongoing and there are numerous family members and friends available, they may wish to set out the food themselves when they are alone and it is convenient for them.

❖ **Find a quiet place close to the hospital room for serving the dinner.** Usually, each hospital unit has a waiting room at the end of the hall. If not too crowded, it can be a perfect place to set up. A donated meal gives more than nutrition when the setting allows family members to gather and unwind.

❖ **Set out and help serve the meal.** In most situations, just set up an informal buffet. Or, you may be asked to leave the food with warming instructions for later.

❖ **Offer to fix up a special plate for anyone who can't leave the bedside or is too upset to eat.** Sometimes folks are too numb or exhausted to serve up even the most delicious meal.

❖ **Offer small portions often.** While someone who is upset may not be able to eat much, small portions of a meal may look more inviting.

CARE TIP	If someone is hospitalized for a long time, family members will likely take turns going home for short periods to rest and clean up. Frozen meals, packed in individual or group portions and stored in the home freezer, can either be brought to the hospital or can be heated up at home. A weary caregiver may love to eat a meal in a private and relaxed place. "There's no place like home."

Cleaning up...

Food can't be left sitting out for long because it will spoil. Someone will need to repackage leftovers and clean up. In hospital waiting rooms, food must be cleaned up pretty quickly for the sake of other families waiting for their loved ones.

❖ **Bring supplies for efficient cleanup.** Consider setting the table with a disposable plastic or paper tablecloth and then when done, wrap up everything in the tablecloth and throw it away.

❖ **Offer to clean up a bit later.** Allow families to remain focused on their loved one by cleaning up afterwards. Be sensitive to those needing time alone or with each other during the mealtime. Offer to give them privacy and to return to clean up in a little while.

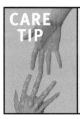 **CARE TIP** | If storage is difficult and food is abundant, consider sharing extra food with hospital staff or other families in distress.

❖ **Repackage the food.** Put leftovers in smaller containers that will easily fit into the refrigerator, freezer, or cooler for a later meal or midnight snack.

❖ **Label repackaged leftovers.** Be sure to date and label the contents of each leftover. If sharing a patient refrigerator in the hospital, put the patient's name and room number on it.

❖ **Clean up the area.** After serving a meal in the hospital, make the waiting room look just like it did before you came. Either take meal-time trash with you or tie it up in bags so that it does not overflow. If visiting at a home, check the trash and empty it if needed.

❖ **Check stored food supply often.** If a number of people are bringing meals into the hospital or to the home, food is likely to accumulate. Rewrap anything that has not been sealed. If using a cooler, be sure to empty out any water and to refill with ample ice or blue ice.

Susan's story

Susan is in the ICU after nearly drowning in an apartment pool and remains in critical condition. Although friends have brought in lots of snacks over the last couple of days, the family has yet to eat a balanced meal since the accident.

The high school band's parent booster club pulls together and plans to deliver the evening meal to the hospital for the whole week. They not only prepare the meal, but also serve it to family members and then clean up afterwards.

❖ **Throw away old food.** Someone needs to go through the cooler or refrigerator and throw away foods that have a tendency to spoil. Check with the family first, before throwing away any foods. They may have been saving something special for that midnight snack.

Types of tasty meals...

In this fast-paced world, not everyone has time to cook from scratch. However, with so many available convenience foods, folks don't have to cook to provide a nutritious and comforting meal.

The sandwich meal...

❖ **Breads** Be creative! Go beyond white sliced bread unless you know that is the family's favorite. Consider bagels, tortillas, pita pocket bread, focaccia bread, and other varieties (wheat, rye, sourdough).

❖ **Sandwich fillings** Tuna, egg, or chicken salad, sliced meats, cheeses, lettuce, tomatoes, red onions, avocado, peanut butter, jelly, jam, etc.

Be sure to keep meats cold and separate from the other ingredients to prevent spoilage.

❖   **Condiments** Mayonnaise, mustards, pickle relish, barbeque sauce, etc.

❖   **Relishes** Pickles, olives, peppers, onions, etc.

❖   **Fruit** Whole fruit is a fresh and healthy treat to accompany the sandwich. Many stores now carry prepared (pre-washed, pre-peeled, pre-cut) fruit in disposable plastic containers.

❖   **Veggies** Like fruit, you can now buy ready-to-eat veggies.

❖   **Chips** Consider individually-sized packaged chips or chips-in-a-can to cut down on storage problems in a hospital room.

❖   **Desserts** Don't forget the cookies, brownies, snack bars, individually pre-packaged puddings, or fruit cups (applesauce, diced fruit).

❖   **Drinks** Consider providing drinks that come in individual portions to make serving easy and to keep storage to a minimum. Think beyond the typical soft drinks and consider juices, teas, flavored waters, or even just plain bottled water.

❖   **Supplies** Bring along knives (for cutting and spreading), paper plates, cups, napkins, plasticware, and storage bags for leftovers. (See "Checklist of Handy Supplies to Bring With the Meal" on page 181.)

The take-out meal...

❖   **Chicken** It comes baked, fried, rotisserie-cooked, and hot or cold. Most major supermarkets, fast-food chains, and delis have these items with all of the side dishes ready to go.

- ❖ **Hamburgers** Hamburgers are the classic fast food. Sometimes it's the perfect choice if you know the family's favorite.

- ❖ **Pizza** Loved by all…devoured by most!

- ❖ **Submarine sandwiches** Find these at fast-food restaurants and most major grocery stores.

8

Mike's story

Mike, a 16 year old, was just in a terrible car wreck. He is in the ICU (Intensive Care Unit) and in critical condition. The family and friends are too distraught to sit down to eat and are even afraid to leave to go to the vending machines.

The basketball coach, a close friend of Mike's family, is also waiting in the ICU. He calls Brian and Jason, Mike's fellow team members, and fills them in on the situation. He asks them to stop off at a nearby submarine sandwich shop and buy a variety of sandwiches that can be shared among the family members and friends in the ICU waiting room.

- ❖ **Ethnic** The list goes on…Chinese, Italian, Mexican, Greek, etc.

- ❖ **Noodle bowls** Imagine…a whole meal in a bowl!

- ❖ **Main-meal salads** You can find all types of salads (pasta, tossed, ethnic, meat, vegetarian).

- ❖ **Catered meals** These can be hot entrees or boxed lunches/meals. Catering companies and most restaurants will provide either carryout or delivery services.

The gift-certificate meal...

Purchase a gift certificate or a coupon book to give to the family. It's great if the business delivers to the hospital or home, but sometimes a family member can run out to a business that is close by to pick up the food when everyone is hungry.

❖ **Provide gift certificates for restaurants or fast-food chains.** Gift certificates can be used whenever needed, either for out-of-town friends or relatives, or when food preparation seems overwhelming. This is the perfect idea for you if you don't like to cook, but still want to do something.

Kevin's story

Kevin's younger sister has just died at home after a long illness. His parents are too exhausted and too much in shock to think about meals for Kevin and his teenaged friends who have come to be with him. A generous neighbor gives Kevin a gift certificate to a local pizza parlor that delivers. The boys order the pizza with plenty to go around for the weary parents as well.

The pre-packaged meal...

❖ **Frozen entrees** You have lots to choose from! Check to be sure that the facility has a freezer and a microwave.

❖ **Ready-to-microwave soups or pastas** More and more of these products are becoming available everyday and they don't require cooling or freezer space. These can be great to have on hand!

❖ **Pre-packaged salads** These come all ready to eat with dressing and croutons. Some even come with cooked, chunked meats.

The home-cooked meal...

Casseroles or other comfort foods make a great main meal for delivering to someone in need. Each part of the United States has its own favorites and flavors including international cuisines.

Sometimes, a couple of people may want to go in on providing a meal and divide up the cooking, delivery, setting up, serving, and cleanup. If many people wish to contribute meals over a period of time, someone may need to coordinate this helping effort.

Find a recipe that is a winner!

❖ **Look through your own favorite family recipes.** Your family may have its own traditional favorites.

❖ **Ask your friends.** Friends who are good cooks will have tried-and-true recipes.

❖ **Surf the Internet.** You'll find tons of recipes on the Internet. Just pull up your favorite search engine and type in key words or key ingredients (chicken dishes, Mexican, casseroles, meatloaf, pasta).

❖ **Check out your favorite cookbooks.** Hiding in all those old cookbooks may be some great recipes that would be perfect.

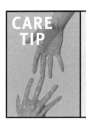

CARE TIP

If you have time, try out the recipe first to see if your family likes it!

Gerry's story

Kathy had just finished making a big pot of her famous chili for Gerry, a co-worker who had fallen in a construction accident. But she didn't know what to do next. Should she deliver it to the hospital? Should she put it in a big plastic bowl? She called Sue, who had volunteered to coordinate meals for Gerry.

Sue knew just what to do. Since Gerry would be in the hospital for another week, Sue told Kathy to freeze the chili into quart-sized freezer bags and hang onto them until Gerry goes home.

Note to helpers...

To be sure all of your support is truly kind,
take a look at Chapter 6, "Caring without offending"
and Chapter 7, "What **to** say, what **not** to say."

Now imagine...

After falling from a ladder, your friend, unconscious and in critical condition, was taken to the hospital. He is taken into surgery immediately. His family anxiously awaits news as they stay in the surgical waiting area.

Before you head off to join them, you check to see what kinds of snacks you already have in your kitchen. You grab fruit, individually-packaged puddings, gum, candy, chips, and a six-pack of soda. Then, you find an extra basket to put them all in. Next, you head to the grocery store and pick up bottles of water, cheese, crackers, and instant soups.

When you arrive at the waiting room, hungry relatives are grateful for the basket of goodies. You visit for a while and leave the basket of food when you go.

Or imagine...

Ken's wife died after a long illness. He never did learn how to cook much and is exhausted after months of caring for his wife. His friends from the community senior center offer to give him a "leg up" by providing meals for a couple of weeks. You organize the meal delivery by scheduling who will bring what when, and by making the necessary reminder calls.

8

In addition, Jim, one of the men from the center, offers to show Ken how to cook some simple meals. Jim's wife died two years ago, and he faced the same problem of not knowing how to cook. In the meantime, he's picked up some pretty good cooking skills that he can pass on to Ken.

Or imagine this...

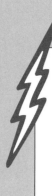

Nine-year-old Sarah, a violinist in a children's orchestra, has been struggling with leukemia. After the initial treatments failed, the parents were told that the final option is a bone marrow transplant. Since the family will need to come up with a large sum of money, the children's orchestra wants to help.

One of the parents, Maria, suggests that the group make and sell breakfast burritos. She has a small licensed catering business and a fabulous recipe from her grandmother. She thinks that they would be a hit for Saturday morning practices. She asks only that the group cover the expense of the ingredients and help with the preparation and sales.

You organize five volunteers to gather at Maria's catering kitchen to make the burritos. They spend the day chopping, cooking, and assembling them. A few volunteers offer to sell the burritos the next day at the Saturday morning practice. Because the group practices in a building at a busy intersection, they even ask a few parents to wear sandwich boards advertising the fresh burritos on the street corner. When the people buying the burritos find out about little Sarah, some of them throw in an extra donation.

Maria's burritos were such a success that the parents have decided to also sell the burritos at evening concerts throughout the year as a continuing fundraiser for Sarah's family.

8

CHAPTER NINE

Giving the perfect gift...

In this chapter you'll find answers to...

- Why is it important to give a gift that counts?

- What are some gift ideas that serve a purpose?

9

Imagine...

You are headed to the hospital to visit a friend. You feel that you ought to bring a gift, but don't have the slightest idea what you should take.

Giving a gift that counts...

Gifts are a concrete way to show that you care, but they can also carry your good wishes. For example, a cozy blanket sends along moments of comfort. A funny disguise or an outrageous hat delivers a bit of laughter. A basket filled with growing bulbs brings with it a hope for each new day.

Some gifts are a way of sharing similar tastes or bringing fresh ideas through books, music, or videos. Some gifts can have a purpose. They can introduce new hobbies like stamp collecting or drawing. An album filled with pictures, stories, and notes can keep the patient connected with his community, while tickets to a much-anticipated event can focus the patient on the future.

9

It's important to choose a gift carefully rather than just give "things." Sometimes, someone who is sick receives so many gifts that the gifts become a burden, requiring organization and storage. In this situation, perhaps it is best to "do something" instead…like offering to run an errand, caring for the family pets, or providing transportation for incoming family. These are gifts, too!

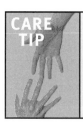

CARE TIP

Remember, a gift need not be an expensive item. A simple sticker, bookmark, or piece of gum tucked into a card shows you care.

Many of the gift ideas are perfect ways for children to express their concern and to learn how to help in a meaningful way. For additional ideas specifically for children, refer to "Visiting ideas for children" on page 66.

This section is chock full of gift ideas to get you started. Maybe you will find the perfect idea here or perhaps these suggestions will inspire your own unique creation.

Gifts that bring a bit of comfort...

Comfort comes in all different forms, with many ways to ease the terrible anxiety and feeling of aloneness that can come with a crisis.

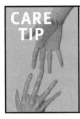

CARE TIP

What's comforting to a baby, young child, teenager, adult, or older person will likely vary. Choose carefully.

❖ **Cozy pajamas** Giving new comfy pajamas or bringing the patient's pajamas from home can add a sense of well-being or comfort to most people.

❖ **Comforters or blankets** These add color and softness to the typically sterile, stark hospital room.

❖ **Pillow from home or a soft new pillow** Hospital pillows are notoriously uncomfortable.

❖ **Decorated or personalized pillowcase** This is simple and easy to do. Use permanent colored markers. Write messages or draw pictures that have special meaning and provide encouragement to the patient.

❖ **Stuffed animals** Who doesn't love a soft, huggable, or funny stuffed animal?

❖ **Lotions** Lotions by themselves can be delightful, and if you know the individual well, offer to rub his or her feet, give a back rub or hand massage.

Gifts of food or beverage...

Special treats sometimes just hit the spot! They can be eaten right away, saved until the patient feels better, or shared with visitors.

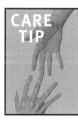 **CARE TIP** Be sure to check with the hospital staff or the family regarding gifts of food or beverages before you bring them (especially for children). Often, people in the hospital are on special diets or are restricted from food or even liquids before procedures or surgery.

9

❖ **Cake in a mug** Just add water and microwave. Voila! You have a cake! Look online for the recipe of your choice.

Basic Instructions:

♦ Choose a regular-size mug (one that holds at least 10 oz. of liquid to the brim).

♦ Put ⅓ cup cake mix (Any flavor and any brand packaged cake mix will do.) in a sealable plastic bag and tie with a ribbon.

♦ If desired, also separately wrap up 1 tablespoon of topping (powdered sugar, chocolate-covered candies, chocolate chips, sprinkles, cinnamon and sugar) to use *after* microwaving the cake.

♦ Insert the packages of ingredients into the mug.

♦ Attach the instructions (next page) to the mug with a ribbon.

—Original Author Unknown

Cake in a Mug

- Empty the cake mix into the mug.
- Add 3 tablespoons water.
- Stir for 30 seconds.
- Microwave on high power for 2 minutes.
- Sprinkle toppings onto the cooked cake.
- Enjoy!

❖ **Cake in a cone** Kids (young and old) love these! This is a fun way to bring a cupcake to someone in the hospital or at home. Again, look online for your favorite variation.

Basic Instructions:

- Use any packaged cake mix. (Yellow cake is usually a safe bet.) Mix according to the cupcake directions.

- Use plain cake cones with the flat bottoms (not sugar cones) and fill each cone ½ full.

- Stand each filled cone into a small cake pan or muffin tin. Follow the package instructions for the correct baking temperature for your area (regular or high altitude). Bake about 15 minutes until the top springs back when pressed.

- Cool and top with your favorite frosting.

- Decorate with your favorite colored candy sprinkles.

- Makes about 30 cones.

—Original Author Unknown

Charlie's story

Charlie has had another corrective surgery resulting from his birth defect, spina bifida. An aunt brings in four mugs filled with the "cake-in-a-mug" recipe for Charlie to share with his family. Dad, who is spending the night with Charlie in his hospital room, isn't sleeping well. At 3 A.M., he microwaves his "cake-in-a-mug" and enjoys the warm snack.

9

- ❖ **Tea/coffee instant mixtures in a mug** This is a fun way to turn a plain mug into something festive.

- ❖ **Specialty coffee drinks** Make it in your own fancy coffee machine at home or stop to pick up one from a local coffee house. Perfect for the family member going on "night watch" or for the much-needed early morning "wake up."

- ❖ **Small fruit baskets** Fruit is a refreshing choice and can be shared with family, visitors, and staff.

- ❖ **Candy & Cookies** Yum! Great for the sweet tooth and for sharing. Caution: Check with the patient for any diet restrictions, and for children, get prior approval from parents.

- ❖ **Bagels** Depending on the topping, bagels can be a healthy choice.

- ❖ **Fast food** Choose his/her favorite kind if you know it. For children, bring fast food with ***prior parental approval.*** Good nutrition may be a concern.

- ❖ **Gum** It's handy any time and fun for the patient to hand out to others.

❖ **Gift certificates** These can be purchased at any favorite food or beverage shop and redeemed at a later date. A gift certificate to a restaurant that will cater to the individual's dietary restrictions would be a fabulous treat!

❖ **Special diet meal** Often people are asked to follow a new diet (low fat, diabetic) following a new medical diagnosis. This can be an overwhelming challenge for someone just coming to grips with the need to make dietary changes. A tasty meal that follows the prescribed diet along with the recipes or a special diet cookbook would be the perfect gift.

Traditional gifts...

These are always welcome and acceptable gifts. They may be just the perfect present.

❖ **Mylar balloons** What a great way to give cheer! Check with the hospital because latex balloons may be restricted due to latex allergy precautions and the danger to children inhaling pieces of popped balloons.

❖ **Flowers or plants** Some people just love flowers and the joy and beauty that they bring! But, you should be aware of some common restrictions. Often, the typical hospital room is too small to handle many flower arrangements. Specialized units like ICU (Intensive Care Unit) or the CCU (Cardiac Care Unit) may not allow these items at all due to the many health-care personnel and monitoring equipment that must fill the patient area. In addition, some hospital units (respiratory, oncology, transplant) may not allow these items to come to the unit due to possible mold, bacteria, or viral contamination that could affect the patient's condition.

❖ **Soaps** Washing hands with a decorative, fresh-smelling soap can counteract the smells of the hospital. Some people, however, cannot tolerate scented soaps, so check first.

❖ **Candles** Candles, now available in unusual shapes, scents, and containers have had a re-lighting of popularity. Caution! Hospitals typically do not allow lighting of candles due to fire precautions. Also, some people cannot tolerate scented candles. Again, check first.

❖ **Stationery** Note cards or writing paper can be used to write thank you notes or just to keep in touch. Include stamps and a pen and this can be the perfect thing for someone who can't be out and about.

❖ **Books** Books with short, separate sections that can be easily read may be best. Often due to stress, side effects of medications, fatigue, nausea, or pain, people cannot concentrate and follow a complicated story line. On the other hand, some people may prefer more complicated books to find a brief mental escape from the crisis.

9

Audio-visual and high-tech gifts...

Today's electronic devices can bring the world to a hospitalized or home-bound patient. Audio-visual gifts not only help make the time fly for the patient, but give the caretaker a break.

❖ **CDs/DVDs** Choose some of the patient's favorite musicians, singers, comedians, or even peaceful nature sounds. These may be especially helpful during sleepless nights or serve as a distraction during painful medical procedures.

❖ **Electronic players with headsets** These small portable devices can be helpful by blocking out the sounds of the hospital world and by providing a distraction during medical procedures.

❖ **Video games** These are popular with kids and many adults.

❖ **Audio books** These can be purchased, rented, or borrowed from the public library.

❖ **Funny audio or video recordings** "Laughter is the best medicine!"

❖ **Popular videos** Please preview the video before giving so you are certain of the content! Consider the child's age, the family's values, and the theme of the video. ***For children, ask the parent's permission.*** The family may have rules regarding the categories of videos their child can see (G, PG, PG 13).

❖ **Classic funny movies** Consider old Laurel and Hardy, Charlie Chaplin, or Three Stooges videos.

❖ **Hobby videos** Ask about the patient's hobbies or interests (cooking, fishing, gardening, sewing, woodworking) and find a video about that subject.

❖ **Travel videos** Is there a favorite place where this patient has traveled? Is the patient planning to travel as soon as he or she is well? Videos for these destinations may be encouraging. ***Caution!*** Unless the patient requests these, do not give videos that will only remind the patient of places she or he can never visit due to declining health.

❖ **Sports videos** Sports fanatics will love these!

❖ **Sports "bloopers"** Even those who are not interested in sports may like these! Who doesn't love watching others look silly?

❖ **Laptops** Laptops travel anywhere—to a hospital, out to the lawn chair in the backyard, or back to the bedroom. Both kids and adults can pass the time away playing computer games or making journal entries. If access to the Internet is available, a bedridden person can link to the world! He or she can check e-mail, talk in chat rooms, shop, search for information about an illness, or learn about anything and everything!

Gifts with a touch of humor...

"Laughter is the best medicine." Even in a difficult situation, humorous gifts are often healing, comforting, and can bring a moment of joy to all.

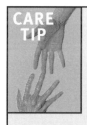

CARE TIP When giving humorous gifts, be careful not to cross the fine line between being funny and being offensive. Carefully consider changes in the patient's health condition. A gift that was funny yesterday may no longer be appropriate if the patient's condition is now critical.

9

❖ **Stickers** Patients can wear them, give them to others, or put them on letters, note cards, or activity books. They can also use them for rewards for the health-care providers who have done a good job. (Giving stickers to health-care providers gives children a healthy way to express thanks. This helps children have some control...they can give them out when they choose.)

❖ **Jokes** You can send, tell, or teach the patient jokes to tell to others.

❖ **Disguises or costume items** Find fake teeth, nose boogers, silly glasses, beards, mustaches, wigs, tattoos, or wax lips at toy, costume, or novelty stores. These are a "must" for kids and teenagers, but also fun and unexpected for adults and older adults as well. Disguises are great for giving visitors or health-care professionals a jolt and giving the patient a good laugh at their reactions!

❖ **Joke items** Again, look in toy, costume, or novelty stores for items such as slimy eyeballs, plastic bugs, fake barf (vomit), fake dog poop, and glow in the dark items. These will provide comic relief and give the individual an amusing outlet. It can reinforce the fact that even in the darkest of times, laughter can be helpful and healthful.

❖ **Funny or unique socks** Give them a chuckle and keep their feet warm at the same time!

❖ **Funny or unique hats** These are great conversation starters.

❖ **Squirt guns** These time-honored toys are winners every time.

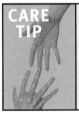

CARE TIP

The items above can provide harmless outlets for playing practical jokes on visitors, hospital staff, and family.

❖ **Letters written on unusual items** Write notes on airplane barf bags, toilet paper on a roll, or on candy wrappers. (Don't forget to send along the candy!)

❖ **Funny cards** Be careful not to cross the fine line between being funny and being offensive.

❖ **Funny cartoon clippings** Scan the newspapers or magazines for funny cartoons or those that are relevant to the person.

❖ **Funny articles, headlines, or photos** Cut these from the paper or magazines.

❖ **Internet items** Print jokes, photos, or stories.

Gifts that fill the time...

❖ **Fingernail polish** Polish fingers or toes...for young or old! Nail polish is a great way to accent an arm or leg cast.

❖ **Manicure sets** Whether the set is just given as a gift or a free manicure is included, this will help fill the time.

❖ **Makeup** Ideal for the teenager! She can use up time practicing.

❖ **Face painting supplies** Perfect for the youngster to paint himself or visitors.

❖ **Playing dough** This can be purchased or homemade. Check online for easy recipes to make playing dough.

❖ **Playing dough kit** Assemble playing dough, cookie cutters, cookie sheet, small rolling pin, and a small spatula. Place in a see-through bag or a box for storing.

❖ **Cookie cutters** Think about including homemade cookies as a treat along with a promise to make cookies together in the future. Not only can the cutters be used for making cookies at a future date, but also as stencils to trace around playing dough or clay.

❖ **Coloring supplies, paper, scissors** Art supplies are great for decorating the room, making cards, or just filling time.

❖ **Colored markers** Perfect for writing on casts or other art projects. Permanent markers won't run if the cast gets wet.

❖ **Activity kits** The choices are limitless! Kits for making necklaces, key chains, belts, etc., can be purchased at most craft stores or you can assemble them yourself. A kit should include everything you need to finish the craft. If you make the kit yourself, put all the supplies in a sealable plastic bag or a decorated shoebox. Include a picture and instructions for the finished craft as an example or let the person be creative.

❖ **Magazines** Magazines with large, colorful pictures and picture books are great for those too tired to concentrate or read. The pictures can also be used for collages or other art projects.

❖ **Games** Travel size may work best.

❖ **Puzzles** It is a challenge to store a puzzle-in-progress in a small hospital room. However, puzzle keepers (available from a puzzle store, puzzle catalog, or online puzzle companies) allow you to roll up a puzzle that is in progress. See page 211 for other ideas.

❖ **Foam target/hoop games** These temporarily attach to the wall or door. These are great for the patient and for visitors. Keep a running scoreboard of visitors who play to determine who's the best!

❖ **Scrapbook** Provide all the supplies so the patient can begin to work on it.

❖ **Collector albums** Start or continue a favorite collection (trading cards, stamps, coins). If you know people who travel, ask them to send cards or coins from different countries to give the collection a jumpstart.

❖ **Playing cards** These are tried and true by themselves or with an offer to teach a new game or play an old one.

❖ **Lap desk** These can be purchased or homemade. An inexpensive lap desk can be made from a four-sided cardboard box. Turn the box so that the smoothest side can be used for the tabletop. To be sure that the tabletop will sit flat on the bed when placed over the patient, make cut outs for the legs. Decorate the lap desk for added flair.

Gifts that keep people in the loop...

❖ **Framed photos or picture albums** These are perfect for including pictures of friends, family, pets, past vacations, or events. Be sure the photos are not painful reminders of permanently lost capabilities (such as an athletic team picture when the patient will never be able to play again). ***Always get permission from the family.***

❖ **Banners with encouragement and signatures** It's better to say, "We miss you," rather than "Get well soon," if this is a long-term or possibly terminal illness.

❖ **Album filled with well wishes, thoughts, and photos** What a fun project for the neighborhood, church, school, place of work, or other organization! This is also a great way to get kids involved.

❖ **Videos of special events** Patients who miss a special event due to the illness might feel more a part of things when they enjoy the video. Consider adding a greeting of "Wish you were here!"

❖ **Audio recordings** Place a voice recorder on the kitchen table and record everyday banter with family, friends, and pets. Before giving the recording to the patient, ***be sure*** to carefully screen for comments that could hurt the patient's feelings or hinder recovery.

❖ **Homemade videos** Create a funny video by gathering a group of friends, family, and pets and start the camera rolling! Record folks saying "Hi," performing a hilarious skit (complete with costumes), or doing other funny things.

❖ **Treats or presents for Fido or other critters** Some patients can hardly wait to get home to their beloved pets. Pet stores are loaded with all kinds of cute toys and treats. They are a great way to help someone sick to look forward to a happy homecoming.

❖ **Jigsaw letter or picture** Glue a letter, picture, or photo to a sturdy piece of cardboard. Cut into puzzle pieces and put into an envelope. The puzzle will need to be assembled before the letter, picture, or photo can be seen.

❖ **Frequent flyer miles.** Often these miles just go to waste. Consider donating your frequent flyer miles to the family so that far away family and close friends can visit. Contact the airlines to find out how to make these arrangements.

Gifts that help folks look to the future...

Often, when people are discouraged by their illness, something that helps to look ahead can make a difference.

❖ **Calendar with a daily joke or cartoon** These can start each day with a grin.

❖ **Tickets to a future event** For the patient who is discouraged, tickets to a favorite event might be a super reward for meeting a goal (getting through a difficult series of treatments, learning new skills, completing rehabilitation exercises).

❖ **Jigsaw puzzles** Bring along a puzzle to work on together each visit. If space is an issue, either purchase a special puzzle storage mat or make one. Buy a piece of heavy felt several inches bigger (on all sides) than the completed puzzle. Assemble the puzzle on the felt. After each visit, roll up the mat with the partially completed puzzle and insert into a large tube. It will be ready and waiting for the next time.

❖ **Read a book aloud.** Find a book you know the patient will enjoy and read a few pages or a chapter at each visit.

❖ **Write a never-ending story.** Send a new episode each week or month. This is a great idea for someone who lives far away and wants to show continuing love and support.

❖ **Seed Kit** Gather a clear glass jar, 5 to 10 cotton balls, and vegetable seeds. Help the patient wet the cotton balls and insert the seeds (1 to 3) into the mound of moist cotton. Keep the cotton moist over time and watch the seeds grow!

❖ **Amaryllis** This tall stunning flower grows quickly from a planted bulb. Include a ruler to track the growth from day to day.

❖ **Tell a never-ending story.** This is perfect for creative folks! Your story will grow with each visit or phone call and the patient will be awaiting each new episode. This is another great idea for those who live far away!

❖ **Leave an inexpensive gift every day or so.** Young or old will look forward to discovering the latest surprise. This is wonderful during a difficult Hanukkah, Christmas, or other holiday season.

❖ **Be a secret pal and leave anonymous little gifts or letters every now and then.** This idea will keep them guessing!

9

❖ **Send postcards** Do you travel to different places or know someone who does? Postcards are available everywhere (airports, drug stores, grocery stores, gift shops). Add a quick note and an interesting stamp and you can bring the world to someone in bed.

❖ **"Warm fuzzy" factory** Find a widemouthed clear plastic bottle, a cardboard box, shoebox, or an empty tissue box, etc. Decorate it with stickers, ribbons, or a collage of photos or pictures from magazines. On brightly colored pieces of paper, write jokes, messages that say something comforting like "You're special because…" or "I like you because…" about the patient. Include instructions that say, "Open one warm fuzzy each day." Of course, likely they will all be opened immediately!

Gifts of your time and service...

In a crisis, people typically want to help by bringing a gift. Sometimes the most valuable gift of all is the gift of helping. Remember, a gift of time and service may be the only thing an individual or family in crisis really wants or needs!

Do something that will make a difference!

❖ **Run the errands.** Find out what needs to be done (laundry picked up, kids taken to activities, grocery shopping).

❖ **Retrieve personal necessities from the home.** These can be comfort items for the patient or items a family member might need at the hospital.

❖ **Watch the family children.** Baby-sit the kids for a few hours or transport them to their ongoing activities (lessons, sports, jobs). If you know the family well, this would be invaluable.

❖ **Mow the lawn.** The individual, family, and neighbors will be so grateful!

❖ **Water the plants/lawn.** The plants and lawn will be thrilled!

❖ **Tend the garden or flower boxes.** Knowing the garden is being cared for can be a big relief.

❖ **Clean the house or have it cleaned professionally.** This should only be done with permission!

❖ **Shovel the snow.** This is a perfect way for kids to help.

❖ **Care for the family critters.** Find out the routine for the pets and keep notes for the family about how they are doing.

❖ **Collect mail and newspapers.** Either put the mail in the house or offer to bring essential mail (bills, cards) to the hospital.

❖ **Make the house looked lived in.** Turn lights off and on. Perhaps, park a car in the driveway.

❖ **Manage the videos.** Bring and return videos to the library or to the video store.

❖ **Maintain a telephone information tree.** With a phone tree, well-wishers can stay in touch without being intrusive. Choose one or more discreet and trusted individuals (with individual/family approval) who can either call with new information or can be called to answers questions. It is difficult for individuals/families in crisis to constantly answer well-meaning questions about how things are going.

9

❖ **Set up and maintain a telephone hotline.** Often, companies, individuals, or non-profit organizations have extra phone lines with voicemail or answering machines that can be donated for a hotline. A family spokesperson or trusted friend can record frequent updates. Those wanting information can simply call the hotline and get updates without needing to bother the family, who is focused on caring for the patient.

Typically, these hotlines are for announcements only and not for leaving messages. The update can tell where to call to leave well-wishes, what support may be needed (such as blood donations), and perhaps best times to visit or call.

❖ **Create and update a social-networking page.** You can keep folks informed by putting together a social-networking page that's devoted to the person who's struggling with a major illness or disability. Of course, be sure to get the patient and family's approval before taking on this project.

❖ **Use an organized web service to create a patient web page.** Web services like *www.CarePages.com* are usually free and make creating and updating a patient's website easy. In addition, they usually are set up with message boards so visitors can leave words of support. They also provide many privacy and safety features that may not be automatic in self-made websites.

❖ **Donate or organize frequent flyer miles.** These miles can make it possible for close friends and family members who live far away to visit and bring encouragement, laughter, and support.

❖ **Coordinate a blood drive.** Contact your local blood donor center. They will give you lots of information and help to set up a successful drive. See "Coordinating a blood drive," page 241.

❖ **Offer to take a walk or do other type of exercise with the patient or with a family member who needs support.** This can be a one-time thing or on an ongoing basis.

❖ **Fix a meal or coordinate ongoing meal preparation and delivery.** Provide a wholesome meal for family members visiting at the hospital or for those staying at home.

❖ **Offer to stay with the patient** while the family member goes home to clean up, sleep, be with other children or family, exercise, or just get away.

❖ **Offer to research information about the illness, drugs, or medical procedures.** Remember, *only pursue this with the family's permission.* They may have chosen a particular treatment path. New information may be confusing, disturbing, or cause them to doubt their decisions. This is particularly hard when the family needs to focus on the patient and see their way through a very grueling time.

❖ **Provide a room at your home** for family members or friends from out of town. For visiting folks who want more privacy, suggest the names of nearby motels or hotels.

❖ **Provide transportation** for out-of-towners. Pick them up from the airport, train, or bus station and get them to the hospital.

9

❖ **Design a web page.** Again, only do this with the patient's or family's permission. This can be great for adolescents! A web page can include photos, fun graphics, and general information about the patient's progress. It can encourage people to write letters or help with their stamp or postcard collection by sending them from wherever people are traveling.

❖ **Ready the home for the patient's return.** This can include cleaning or airing the home, opening curtains, cleaning or stocking the refrigerator, or making simple repairs. Or, perhaps adjustments (wheelchair ramp, bathroom bar, hand-held shower) need to be made to the home for the patient's changed condition.

❖ **Offer your professional skills.** You may have special knowledge (insurance, legal, health care, disability, career counseling) that you can directly share or use to help the family obtain resources.

Gifts for folks staying close by at the hospital...

Imagine what it is like to stay in the hospital with a loved one, day in and day out. What a fine opportunity this is to give a gift that shows you care and that you are concerned about the caregiver as well.

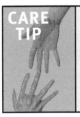

CARE TIP

Look through the miscellaneous collections of shampoos and lotions that you have brought home from motels or hotels on trips. These are the perfect size for this kit.

Personal Care Kit
(For the person staying close by at the hospital)

- ☐ Breath mints
- ☐ Gum
- ☐ Toothbrushes
- ☐ Toothpaste
- ☐ Dental floss
- ☐ Mouthwash
- ☐ Lip balm
- ☐ Liquid body soap
- ☐ Wash cloth (pack separately in a small re-sealable plastic bag for when wet)
- ☐ Hand towel
- ☐ Razor
- ☐ Shaving cream
- ☐ Shampoo
- ☐ Conditioner
- ☐ Comb or brush
- ☐ Deodorant
- ☐ Lotion
- ☐ Tissues
- ☐ Packaged hand wipes
- ☐ Feminine products
- ☐ Sewing kit
- ☐ Plastic trash bag for dirty clothes
- ☐ Sleep mask
- ☐ Ear plugs

Put the above supplies together in a plastic container or bag.

9

Comfort Kit

- ☐ Stationery & pen
- ☐ Postage stamps
- ☐ Address or email lists (from the neighborhood, church, work, clubs, teams) for keeping in touch
- ☐ Blank journal book
- ☐ Current magazines
- ☐ Uplifting or entertaining book
- ☐ Deck of playing cards
- ☐ Pad of paper
- ☐ Puzzle or crossword book
- ☐ Gum or breath mints
- ☐ Snacks
- ☐ Healthy bottled beverages
- ☐ An assortment of coins or dollar bills for phone calls, vending machines, or parking

Put the above supplies together in a plastic container or bag.

Gifts for the professional caregivers...

Families are never obligated to give gifts of thanks to caregivers. Still, people often want to make a small gesture to show their appreciation for the care of their loved one. Perhaps some of these suggestions may fit your situation.

❖ **Notes or cards** This is a gift from the heart. The professional caregiver will remember this long after the paycheck has been spent.

❖ **Recognition cards** Most hospitals have formal recognition programs that make it possible for family and friends to say "thanks" to employees for their efforts. Sometimes these are posted for all to see.

❖   **Letters to managers** What a great way to say "thanks" and make a difference for an exceptional employee. Often, the letter will be placed in the employee's personnel file and can impact the employee's evaluation.

❖   **Food for staff** This is a nurturing warm way to say "thanks" to a group.

- ◆   Coffee/teas

- ◆   Cookies

- ◆   Candy

- ◆   Bagels

- ◆   Popcorn (pre-popped, flavored, microwaveable)

- ◆   Fruit tray or basket

- ◆   Vegetable tray

- ◆   Cheese and cracker tray

- ◆   Relish tray

- ◆   Deli-style sandwich tray (breads, meats, cheeses, lettuce, sliced tomatoes, condiments)

- ◆   Gift certificates for pizza delivery These can be used by a particular shift or by the entire floor or department.

❖   **Donation to a hospital fund in an employee's or department's name**
This is a great way to recognize the work that a group provides.

9

❖ **Contributions for the hospital unit** This is a good way to contribute to the work of a unit/department.

◆ Magazine subscriptions for the waiting rooms

◆ Videos

◆ Books

◆ Small stuffed animals (new) to be given to children

◆ Toys (yo-yos, activity kits, games, puzzles)

Note to helpers...

To be sure all of your support is truly kind,
take a look at Chapter 6, "Caring without offending"
and Chapter 7, "What *to* say, what *not* to say."

Now imagine...

Your elderly neighbor has fallen and broken her hip. She is discouraged, as her doctor has told her that she will need to spend several months recovering in a nursing home before she will be able to go home. You want to give her a gift that will let her know that her neighbors are thinking about her and remembering her. You ask the neighborhood children to help you make a big colorful banner for everyone to sign. You supply the big roll of paper and lots of colorful markers, and let the kids create the design. Then you have them take it around for everyone to write their messages of encouragement. As your neighbor moves into the nursing home, you make sure that it gets mounted on the wall where she can see it.

9

Or imagine...

Your 10-year-old nephew is home from the hospital after being hit by a car while riding his bike. He is in quite a bit of pain and needs to stay quiet, but is bored. You want to give him a number of little gifts that will help distract him from the pain and also keep him entertained. You head to the nearest discount store and find a small model airplane, a simple paint-by-numbers kit, and a simple jigsaw puzzle that pictures his favorite animal. You wrap up each separately and mark each to be opened on a given day (Monday, Wednesday, Friday).

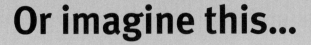

Or imagine this...

Your adult child has been chronically ill for several years, unable to work for weeks at a time. Since you live across the country, you can't visit often. However, your job entails quite a bit of world travel. You decide you will send her postcards from your many destinations. You start things off by sending her an album for her collection with the promise that the postcards will begin arriving soon. Your travels take on new meaning as you search for unique and fun postcards that will bring a needed smile.

CHAPTER TEN

Writing the right note...

In this chapter you'll find answers to...

- What are some easy steps for writing an encouraging note or letter?

- How do you write a sympathy note that is heartfelt?

10

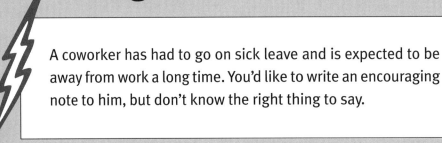

Imagine...

A coworker has had to go on sick leave and is expected to be away from work a long time. You'd like to write an encouraging note to him, but don't know the right thing to say.

Notes that say you care...

Notes have different purposes. Just like gifts, notes can deliver a sense of comfort, affection, encouragement, or compassion. They can also bring a smile and a bit of hope.

Notes will vary. The closer you are to someone, the less formal the note will be. A note to a dear friend, for example, will be more casual than a note to an acquaintance. Also, consider the age of the person. A note to a child will be worded more simply than a note to an adult.

Be respectful of religious beliefs and cultural differences when writing a note. Do not impose your personal values on someone going through a crisis. This is a time to *demonstrate* caring. See "What *to* say, what *not* to say" on page 147.

Sometimes, writing a note can be tough, especially if you don't know where to begin. Here are step-by-step suggestions and easy-to-follow examples to make writing notes or letters of encouragement or sympathy a bit easier.

10

A note of encouragement – step by step...

A note of encouragement should be just a few sentences. Feel free to use the examples below or create your own versions. Of course, don't use the quotation marks ("") that we use in the following examples when you are writing your note.

❖ **Open with the person's name or nickname.**

◆ "Dear Nicki,"

◆ "Hi there, Charlie!"

❖ **Begin with a greeting, just as if you were there in person.**

- ◆ "How are things going?"

- ◆ "How are you doing?"

- ◆ "What's up?"

❖ **Acknowledge that you know what has happened.**

- ◆ "I heard you had surgery."

- ◆ "Sarah told me about your accident."

- ◆ "I was so sorry to hear about the tough news you got from your doctor."

- ◆ "I heard you're having a rough time."

❖ **Continue with a comment about the person's situation.**

- ◆ "How hard this must be for you."

- ◆ "What a rotten deal."

- ◆ "I wish this hadn't happened to you."

- ◆ "How awful."

- ◆ "This is so unfair."

❖ **Include an encouraging comment.**

- ◆ "Hang in there!"

- ◆ "Know that I am thinking about you."

- ◆ "I'm looking forward to seeing you soon."

- ◆ "I can hardly wait to see you back at church."

- ◆ "We've really missed you at softball practice. It'll be great to have you back in the game."

- ◆ "I'm wishing you only the best."

- ◆ "I hope you have a steady recovery."

❖ **End with a kind closing.**

- ◆ "Sincerely,"

- ◆ "Your friend,"

- ◆ "Fondly,"

- ◆ "Love,"

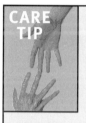

CARE TIP

Be careful not to fill your letter with alternative health care suggestions. You might say simply, "If you are interested in learning about possible treatments, I can scan the Internet or review the literature," or "I know someone who had success with _____ (type of) treatment. If you are interested in more information or want to talk to that person, give me a call."

10

Sample note of encouragement

Dear Emily,

How are you? We missed you at the garden club meeting last week. That was where I heard that you broke your hip and that you're living with your son while you recover. I bet you can hardly wait to get home to your garden and all your bird feeders. Well, keep on getting better so you can get back to garden club next month.

Your fellow flower lover,
Jane

A letter of encouragement — longer and newsier...

A letter of encouragement stretches the note into a lengthier version, perhaps filled with a funny story, the latest news, or a memory you have shared.

❖   **Open with the person's name or nickname.**

❖   **Begin with a greeting, just as if you were there in person.**

❖   **Acknowledge that you know what has happened.**

❖   **Include an encouraging comment.**

❖   **Continue with more encouragement and perhaps what you will do to help.** *Only* include a promise to help if you are sure you will follow through.

❖   **Expand the note into a letter.**

   ◆   Tell a funny story. Here are some ways to start the story.

      ●   "Let me tell you something funny that happened the other day."

      ●   "You should have seen what happened to Amy."

   ◆   Give the latest news or tell about something interesting that has happened to someone you both know. Again, here are some starters.

      ●   "Let me fill you in about what's been going on at work."

      ●   "The skit at the church's picnic was hilarious."

- "Hey, you should see the neighbor's new dog."

- "Remember Sam from the team? He retired and moved up to Alaska to fish!"

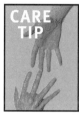

CARE TIP

Remember, this is a letter of encouragement. Keep your news upbeat. Do not tell about your own aches and pains. Avoid gruesome stories or critical comments about others.

◆ Recall a special moment you have shared in the past. Try starting with something like this.

- "The other day I was thinking about our camping trip to the desert."

- "Remember when we laughed so hard we fell over?"

- "We sure were troublemakers at school. We drove Mrs. Harris nuts!"

❖ **Add a final encouraging comment.**

◆ "Just remember, you're in my thoughts and prayers every day."

◆ "Here's a hug for you."

◆ "Feel my arms around you."

◆ "Have a speedy recovery." (Write this *only* if a recovery is possible.)

◆ "Get well soon." (Again, use this *only* if a recovery is possible.)

◆ "Don't give the nurses too much trouble!"

10

❖ **End with a kind closing.** Remember, in the letter you write, don't add quotation marks ("").

- ◆ "My best to you,"

- ◆ "See you soon,"

- ◆ "Thinking of you,"

- ◆ "All my love,"

- ◆ "Love ya,"

- ◆ "You go, girl/guy!" (Or, use any current popular phrasing that is encouraging.)

❖ **Slip something that's interesting, uplifting, or humorous into the envelope.**

- ◆ Poem

- ◆ Article from a newspaper or magazine

- ◆ Cartoon

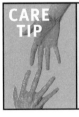 **CARE TIP** Over time, make or purchase nice cards or notepaper to have on hand when you need them. Also, consider collecting encouraging articles, sayings, poems, or jokes to include in an encouraging letter.

Sample letter of encouragement

Hey Buddy,

It was good to see you last Thursday. I know you have a long recovery ahead and I'm sorry you are so bummed out. Who wouldn't be? I'm just glad you're still around after that fall! Good friends are really hard to find. Count on me to come by once a week after work to give you a bad time and to make sure you do that rehab. Hey, we'll do it together and maybe I'll get back in shape, too.

I sure missed you this weekend on our hunting trip. I needed you there to watch my back. Bill tripped and nearly blew me away. Plus, his cooking is lousy. We all sure missed your great stew. Keep on working with all those exercises and you'll be back ready to hunt next year.

Hang in there,
Stu

P.S. Check out the cartoon. Doesn't the fellow look like our clumsy friend Bill?

10

The sympathy note — step by step...

A sympathy note is written to someone grieving after the death of a loved one. While most notes of this kind are sent immediately after someone's death, others will arrive much later as the news of the loss travels. Sympathy notes are a gift in themselves in that they can be read over and over, even years after the loss. Sometimes, sympathy notes can share stories or unknown bits of information about the loved one, giving comfort during a time of sadness.

❖ **Open with a greeting.**

◆ "Dear Bertha,"

❖ **Begin with words of sorrow.**

◆ "I was so sorry to hear about your father's death."

◆ "I am sorry about your loss."

◆ "I'm so sorry to hear that Mark has passed on."

◆ "The loss of your husband touches so many of us."

◆ "I have just heard about Margie's death."

◆ "I hurt for you."

❖ **Make a special comment about the service if you were able to attend.**

◆ "The service was really special."

◆ "It was clear from the picture display that he loved you all."

◆ "I had never heard some of those stories that people shared about her. It was obvious she loved to have fun."

◆ "The music you chose for the service was beautiful. Knowing Bill, he would have loved it."

❖ **Continue with how you are affected by the loss.**

◆ "I will miss Maria so much."

◆ "It hurts so much to think that Dwight won't be here to tell us funny stories."

◆ "Work will be such a drag without Jan."

◆ "Coffee just won't taste the same without Dave there to give me the latest weather report."

- "I can't imagine the neighborhood without Martin walking his dog every evening."

❖ **Include the memory of an endearing quality or shared moments with the deceased.**

- "I will always remember how much Elliot loved to read a mystery and had to tell me the ending before I had a chance to read it."

- "I treasure the times we spent together."

- "I remember when Harriet and I threw that surprise party for you."

- "I smile when I think about Helen laughing at the baby's antics."

- "I will always remember the time when Richard and I did the walk-a-thon together."

- "Just thinking about Anne gives me a warm feeling."

- "Jack always spoke so highly of you."

- "Sonny would always tell about the time when you ran the car into the garage door. He would laugh and laugh."

- "Lyla was the most frequently requested waitress here at the restaurant."

- "James stopped for a doughnut here every morning."

- "Virginia was so kind to my dog every morning when she walked by. She always gave her a little treat."

❖ **Add warm words, wishes, or offers.**

- "Just know that you are in my heart and prayers."

- "Remember, God is with you and has His arms around you."

10

- "We care so much about you."

- "Feel our arms around you."

- "God loves you so much."

- "I hope that the wonderful memories of your life with Frank will bring you comfort and peace."

- "I hope that knowing that Minnie is now with her loving God brings you some peace."

- "I'll bring dinner by on Monday evening."

- "I will call you in a couple of weeks so we can all get together."

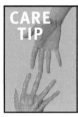

CARE TIP

Remember, do not offer to call, visit, or help unless you are sure you will be able to follow through!

❖ **End with a kind closing.** Again, don't use quotation marks ("") in your sympathy note.

- "Love,"

- "With love,"

- "Affectionately,"

- "Fondly,"

- "Prayerfully,"

- "Warmly,"

Sample sympathy note

Dear Corrine,

Mark's passing is so very sad and will affect so many people. The funeral service was a real tribute to Mark. I especially loved how your children shared their special memories of their dad. You must be so proud that you and Mark raised such a beautiful family.

Work just won't be the same without Mark's funny jokes and stories to start our day. I remember the time when he was mimicking the boss and didn't realize the boss was right behind him. Mark kept us all in stitches. I feel so lucky to have known him.

Please know that you are in my heart. I'd like to meet you for a cup of coffee after everything settles down.

Warmly,
Jean

10

Note to helpers...

To be sure all of your support is truly kind, take a look at Chapter 6, "Caring without offending" and Chapter 7, "What *to* say, what *not* to say."

Now imagine...

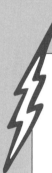

Your best friend's mother has passed away, so you want to send a special sympathy letter. Rather than just buying the typical sympathy card with pre-printed wishes, you choose a nice blank card. You write your own thoughts remembering a time when her mother took both of you on a picnic to the mountains years ago.

Or imagine...

Your coworker has had to take an extended sick leave. Because you don't know the coworker well, but want him to know you are thinking of him, you send an encouraging note that is simple and brief.

Or imagine...

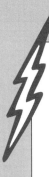

Your Great Aunt Elizabeth fell and broke her hip. She's had a rough time in the hospital and now is discouraged because she cannot go home, but must stay in a rehabilitation center for at least a couple of months.

You live far away and will not be able to visit. You decide to send an encouraging letter every week to keep her looking ahead and to lift her spirits. You make a special effort to fill her in on all of your children's antics. In one of the weekly letters you include recent photos of the kids. In another letter, you include pictures they have drawn. In yet another, you send along your children's notes of well wishes.

10

PART IV
Bigger efforts...

CHAPTER ELEVEN

Coordinating a blood drive...

In this chapter you'll find answers to...

- Why is blood such an important gift?

- What are the steps for putting together a successful blood drive?

- How can you build a blood drive that does more than just bring in the pints?

- What else is important to do after the blood drive?

11

Imagine...

Your neighbor was given lots of blood following an accident. You want to help replace the pints he needed since you've heard that the community blood supply is low. You'd like to help with a blood drive, but you don't know where to start.

Blood — a gift of life...

A donation of blood is such an invaluable gift since healthy people are the only resource. Should someone you know be given blood or need blood on an ongoing basis, a blood drive is a perfect opportunity to help in a very meaningful way.

Organizing and hosting a blood drive will do at least three wonderful things. It will not only help the individual needing the blood, but it will also help replenish the community blood supply. As a bonus, it will pull folks together as a community as they come to help in a common cause.

But, if your time is limited and you cannot host a blood drive, you can still make a huge difference. Let people know with flyers, letters, e-mails, or text messages that your friend or relative needs blood. Simply refer them to the hospital or donation center to give blood in the person's name.

In this chapter, you'll find tips for how to make your blood drive a very friendly and successful event. Don't forget to check online for additional information.

What a potential donor may want to know...

Most people have never given blood and may have many questions and concerns. Actually, only a small fraction of people ever donates blood. Concerned folks will likely want to know:

❖   Even just one pint of whole blood can help save up to three patients.

❖   Donating blood is safe. You cannot get HIV or AIDS from donating blood.

11

❖   Giving blood only takes an hour of your time, with the actual procedure lasting no more than ten minutes.

❖   Your body will replace the blood volume (plasma) within 48 hours. It will take about six to eight weeks for your body to completely replace the red blood cells you donated. (www.redcross.org)

❖   People who still have concerns or more questions should go to the Internet, searching websites for the local blood donor center, local hospitals, or the American Red Cross (www.redcross.org). These websites will have up-to-date information on giving blood.

Planning the blood drive...

There's a lot to do ahead of time to be sure that you have a great blood drive.

Finding a place to hold your blood drive...

❖   **Check with the hospital where the patient is receiving care.** Do they collect blood at their own donation center or do they have a mobile blood drive operation? If not, the hospital may refer you to a local donor organization to assist you in hosting a blood drive.

❖   **Ask at the local blood donation center.** In a small town, there may be only one donor organization or just the community hospital that collects blood. Larger cities may have several blood donor organizations that collect and provide blood for several area hospitals.

❖   **Check the Internet.** Search for local blood donation centers in your area. Also, the American Red Cross website has lots of helpful information about giving blood and coordinating a blood drive.

❖ **Determine the donation site.** Be sure the site (hospital, donor center, worksite, church, school, community center, service organization) has a large room, excellent lighting, electrical outlets, plenty of parking spaces, and bathrooms. Check with the blood donation center for additional requirements.

David's story

David, a 40-year-old man with cancer, needed several pints of blood to strengthen him for an upcoming surgery. During the procedure and in the days that followed, he required 15 more units of whole blood. A buddy in his small farming community organized a blood drive at the larger county hospital. The successful blood drive not only provided blood for David, but also helped to refill the community supply.

❖ **Choose the best date and time to get the most donors.** If the blood drive is held at the worksite, choose a time convenient to the company and its employees. Perhaps the company will allow employees to go during their work time. Other companies may prefer that the workers go during their lunch break or before or after work.

If the blood drive is held in the community, consider weekend days if the donor center can provide support staff. Remember, the blood not only has to be drawn, but must be processed, so a lab must be available.

Getting the word out...

Numbers count. The more folks who know about your blood drive, the more pints you will get. And, that's the goal!

11

Publicity is key!

Careful planning is crucial for a successful blood drive. Pull together a number of folks to help.

❖ **Get pre-made flyers from the blood donor center.** Most donor centers will provide ready-made flyers and then you just write in the date, time, and location.

❖ **Design your own flyers and posters.** In some cases, you may want to design your own flyers and posters so you can highlight the patient's urgent need for blood. Artistic people with graphic design skills or just "a good eye" can be helpful here. Think about creating a slogan ("Pints for Pete," "Blood for Bob") to inspire folks to donate. Don't forget contact names and numbers. If you choose to create your own flyers and posters, be sure to get final approval from the donor center.

❖ **Ask the family first!** If you create a flyer with any information or photos about the person needing blood, be sure to ask the individual or family to review the material first. Many families might not be comfortable with flyers circulating with their personal information or photos.

❖ **Copy flyers and posters.** Some businesses are willing to donate copying services for a good cause.

❖ **Find places willing to display flyers and posters.** Some people either have connections with businesses or are willing to go door-to-door to the businesses, schools, churches, or service organizations, etc. that may have a tie to the individual needing blood.

❖ **Deliver flyers or posters.** Though some people aren't artistic, they can drive and deliver.

❖ **Use the phone.** Get a list and start calling. Find a key person within each organization or group (neighborhood, work, school, service organization, sports team) to spread the word.

❖ **Tell everyone you see.** Keep flyers in hand as you go along during the day so you can give them to folks who are interested.

❖ **Publicize using high technology.** If a website has been created for the patient, just add the blood drive information. If one does not already exist, find someone who can develop one.

Don't forget the power of e-mails and FAX-blasts. Both are terrific ways to quickly get out the information.

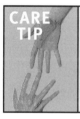

| CARE TIP | Don't limit the blood drive to just the folks who know the patient. You'll be surprised to find that many people will show up for a good cause. |

Who should know?

❖ **Relatives** While the immediate family may seem like a reasonable source, they may be too overwhelmed and exhausted to give blood. Sometimes, relatives beyond the immediate family may be a better choice.

❖ **Neighbors** When neighbors learn about a crisis, they will very likely want to help. If the individual or family has moved around, don't forget to notify people in their old neighborhoods.

11

- ❖ **Schools** Consider notifying not only the school where the children are presently attending, but also schools where they have attended in the past (elementary, middle school, high school). Often, the PTA, PTO, or PTSA is well organized and will have a contact person who can distribute information and coordinate food donations as well. In addition, schools usually have newsletters and websites that are available to students and families.

- ❖ **Churches, synagogues, and temples** Often people have attended or have had connections to more than one place of worship. Think about contacting these organizations. Religious organizations also come with built-in paid staff and volunteers who can help notify people through worship service announcements, bulletins, newsletters, committees, e-mails, and websites.

Chuck's story

Chuck has played on the same softball team for five years. When he heard about David's illness, he spoke with the rest of the softball team. They enthusiastically agreed to be a part of the blood drive in some way. Chuck contacted David's buddy, who was coordinating the blood drive with the hospital, to see how they could all help.

Even though some players did not meet the requirements for giving blood, they volunteered to drive others the 75 miles to the hospital. Two others agreed to contact David's neighbors to let them know about the blood drive. On the big day, several team members, famous for their chili and cornbread, provided a meal for the donors before they headed back home.

❖ **Athletic teams** From baseball to shuffleboard, from women to men, from kids to adults, contact any and all teams where a family member might have been or is connected.

❖ **Activity clubs** It's amazing how people spend their time! Ask about any clubs that the individual, family, or friends attend (book, camera, fishing, quilting, cards, computer, bird watching, speaking clubs).

❖ **Professional organizations** Ask about any work-related groups to which the individual or family may be connected (unions, lawyers, nurses, journalists, educators, physicians, musicians).

❖ **Worksites** Past or present worksites where the family has been connected might have people ready, willing, and able to give blood, pass the word, or volunteer to assist with the blood drive in some way. Larger companies usually have bulletin boards, newsletters, or websites where information can be posted.

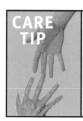

CARE TIP

Remember, do not pressure people to donate blood! Many people may have very personal reasons (such as sexual histories) for why they cannot and should not donate blood!

11

❖ **Service organizations** Usually, service organizations exist to help and are especially responsive when a member needs their support. They often help non-members as well. Also, service organizations probably have a telephone tree system, a website, and a newsletter for reaching their members.

Scheduling for success!

The goal is to end up with the most pints of blood possible. Be sure to fill your time slots with folks who can actually donate blood. While many are willing, not all will meet the requirements.

The rules for donating blood are constantly changing and may vary from place to place. Most donation centers have restrictions for illness, tattoos, piercings, foreign travel, blood counts, blood pressure, etc. Unfortunately, many folks sign up to give blood, not knowing that their blood can't be accepted.

Be sure to get as many qualified people as possible to sign up.

❖ **Arrange to have at least two schedulers.** To be sure someone is always available to take calls, find folks who are close to a phone and willing to schedule individuals for the blood drive. These schedulers will need to keep in close contact with each other to avoid double booking.

❖ **Determine the number of donors that can be scheduled per hour.** Many staff are required to make a blood drive go smoothly. The number of employees available will determine the number of donors per hour. Some staff will insert the needles and collect the blood, while other employees will take histories or process the blood.

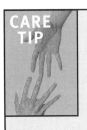

CARE TIP

When people give blood for someone, they often assume that their pint will go directly to that person. But because of the blood matching process, it may not. In that case, your gift of life will go to someone else, and your pint will be credited to your friend or relative and help reduce blood transfusion costs.

❖ **Always allow for a few drop-ins.** Regardless of how well you plan, some folks will still drop in at the last minute. Don't turn away a good donor! Anticipate this.

❖ **Provide blood donation rules ahead of time.** Create a flyer, get one from the donation center, or refer interested donors to the blood donation center for more information. This is *essential*. Many people sign up for blood drives only to discover on the day of the drive that they have a condition or a situation that prohibits them from donating. If folks can refer to the rules ahead of time, they will know if they are eligible.

❖ **Schedule only the donors who are familiar with the rules.** This way, you can be pretty sure that the time slot is filled with someone who is eligible. Of course, you may still have people who end up sick, have low blood pressure, or some other sudden issue on the day of the drive. This can't be helped.

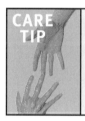

CARE TIP

> Avoid letting people share their personal past or their medical histories when they call to schedule. Instead, schedulers should encourage them to call the blood donor center or hospital for further information.

❖ **Give frequent donors information about transferring or crediting their donation to the patient.** Some people routinely give blood to a particular blood donor center or through a special worksite donation program. However, they can usually switch their typical donation and give blood in the name of a specific person.

❖ **Use the "Blood Drive Schedule" form on page 309 for scheduling.** This form will help you collect the essential information for reminder calls and signing in people the day of the drive.

11

❖ **Consider recruiting for bone marrow donors during the blood drive.**
A blood drive can be the perfect time to also inform people about the
critical need for bone marrow donors. Many blood-related diseases
(leukemia, aplastic anemia) are treated with a bone marrow transplant.
Check with the donor center to see if they will provide information
about this program and perhaps recruit bone marrow donors during
the blood drive.

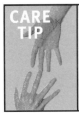

CARE TIP Some folks will not be able to give blood. However, people who
can't donate can help with many other jobs (driving donors,
babysitting, providing refreshments) that will make a blood
drive successful.

❖ **Remind people about their promise to donate blood or help with
the drive.** With their busy lives, people appreciate a reminder call. Be
ready with directions to the donor site.

Getting the blood drive room ready...

Set up the room long before anyone walks in the door.

❖ **Gather a crew of helpers.** Many hands make the work go faster.

❖ **Open up the building.** Don't forget to get a key or the lock combination
so you can enter the building, especially on a weekend or evening when
regular employees aren't around.

❖ **Turn on the heat or air-conditioning.** Be sure the temperature of the
room is comfortable.

❖ **Turn on the lights.** Good lighting for the blood drive is essential for those trying to find veins in arms.

❖ **Set up tables and chairs.** The blood donor center will likely bring in special chairs for folks giving blood. Talk to the donor center for the number of tables that will be needed for their work. Other tables and chairs will be necessary for registration and other stations manned by volunteers.

❖ **Gather other supplies.** As you think of your supply list, consider what you want to accomplish and the activities that will be happening throughout the drive. For example, nametags will make it easier for everyone to connect and chat each other.

If you plan on making posters for the patient, you will need the paper and markers to make it colorful. If you are going to have a babysitting area, you will need things to keep the children entertained.

The blood donation center will usually provide juice and cookies, but if you are going to provide home-baked goods, then decide if you need additional cups, plates, plasticware, or napkins.

❖ **Arrange for a childcare area.** If you expect donors or helpers will need to bring children, make arrangements for a babysitting room close by. Don't forget to advertise that childcare is available.

11

Making the event great...

Holding a blood drive to get lots of units of blood is wonderful. But, perhaps, you'll want to do some extra things that will not only bring in donors, but will also help the community keep the family in mind.

Blood Drive Supply List

☐ Name tags

☐ Laptop computer or pads of paper for collecting address information

☐ Sign-up sheets for other volunteer opportunities (animal care, meals, driving to appointments, yard care)

☐ Extension cords for lights, laptop, or other unanticipated electrical needs

☐ Additional lighting

☐ Colored pencils and markers for making signs and posters

☐ Large paper or poster board for large cards, posters, or signs

☐ Juices

☐ Juice dispenser

☐ Coffee pots

☐ Bottled water

☐ Cups

☐ Cookies

☐ Napkins

☐ Plasticware

☐ Video player for childcare area

☐ Puzzles, paper, crayons, books, movies for children in the babysitting area

Paying attention to the details...

There are a lot of little things that you can do to make a big difference on the day of the blood drive. Make the event friendly and fun.

❖ **Greet folks at the door.** A friendly greeting is always helpful if people are a bit nervous about donating blood. It's also helpful to show people the way to the donation room, especially if the building is large and the donors are not familiar with the layout.

❖ **Register folks as they come in.** Keep track of all helpers as well as all blood donors. This list will be nice to give to the family.

❖ **Provide refreshments.** While the donation center usually provides store-bought cookies and juice, you can make the event even better with homemade items. This is a great opportunity for bakers to contribute, especially if they are not able to donate blood. Keep someone at the refreshment station to remind people to have a bite to eat after giving blood.

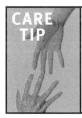

CARE TIP

Remember, people who give blood need to drink lots of liquid to rehydrate. Water or juices are best since caffeine drinks (coffee, tea, soda) tend to dehydrate the body.

❖ **Provide transportation for those who can't drive.** Some of your best donors may need a ride. Don't forget them.

❖ **Design a big card or poster for the patient.** Assign someone be at a table with paper and markers ready to encourage people to write and draw cheerful messages.

11

❖ **Provide childcare.** Responsible older teenagers or adults can watch children in a separate room while parents are donating blood. Think about having the children color pictures or cards for the individual or family. You also might want to provide a *short* G-rated video to also entertain the kids.

❖ **Shovel snow at the blood drive site.** Weather happens! If snow is threatening, be sure to have a crew ready to shovel walks, plow the parking lot, spread salt, and help people into the building if the ground is slippery.

❖ **Keep people dry during a rainstorm.** Don't let bad weather get in the way. Have people ready with umbrellas to walk people into the building. This is a great job for teenagers.

❖ **Say "goodbye" and thank all donors and volunteers as they leave.** Have someone stationed at the door to thank everyone for helping to make the blood drive a success.

Building additional community support...

During a blood drive, people may want to know about other ways they can help the family. Be ready with information about the family's needs, but be sure you have checked with the family first.

❖ **Information table** Have folks available who tell people what is needed (delivery of meals to the hospital or home, pet care, frequent flyer miles, home cleaning, prayer) and who can answer specific questions.

❖ **Sign-up sheets** Have sign-up sheets ready for folks who want to help (flight miles, meals, yard, pet care). Get contact numbers so that after the blood drive, volunteers cannot only call to give further details, but can also confirm time and place.

❖ **Flyer** Prepare a flyer for people to take home. Include a list of the family's needs and numbers to call to sign up.

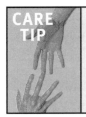

CARE TIP

If the family has medical bills piling up, consider adding a fundraiser (carnival, bake sale, car wash) to the blood drive.

❖ **T-shirts** These are popular with kids and new technology makes them easy to design. A T-shirt that is designed for the blood drive can be worn by the volunteers the day of the blood drive and be sold for a slight profit to help with the family expenses.

❖ **Mugs** Again, personalized mugs can be a simple fundraiser and will bring a reminder of the individual or the event with every sip.

Remembering the family with a keepsake...

Be sure that folks remember the patient and the family long after the blood drive. Giving every volunteer and donor a simple keepsake not only keeps the family in their thoughts, but also builds community spirit. Be sure to check with the individual or family and get their approval first!

❖ **Refrigerator magnet** A homemade magnet with the slogan from the blood drive ("Pints for Pete," "Blood for Bob," "You made a difference!") will be an ongoing "thank you."

❖ **Pens** These days, it's pretty easy to get pens imprinted with a simple slogan.

❖ **Ornaments** A homemade ornament can be put on a Christmas tree each year or hung year round. It can be a great annual reminder of the community's love and spirit.

11

❖ **Candy** Choose a candy that ties in a message. For example, attach a note that says, "You're a lifesaver!" to a package of Lifesavers® candy.

Or, put several Hershey's Candy Kisses® or Hershey's Candy Hugs® in a little cloth bag with the message, "Today, you gave the sweet gift of life."

Following up after the blood drive...

A really successful blood drive isn't over the day of the event. Folks who helped, even those who didn't personally know the patient prior to the blood drive, will feel like they've made a difference and that they've been part of an important effort. Design a simple flyer, e-mail, or newsletter as a quick way to fill everyone in. Phone calls work, too.

Keep people updated and build community spirit.

❖ **Congratulate and thank all those who helped.** A genuine thank you acknowledges and reinforces volunteers' efforts.

❖ **Let people know the results of the blood drive.** Share the final number of pints that were collected and the tally for any other donations received that day.

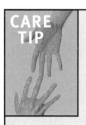

CARE TIP

A website, social-networking page, or telephone hotline about the patient is a great way to pass along results of a blood drive, fundraisers, the patient's condition, or future events. Of course, always check with the family before adding any new information.

❖ **Keep people updated on the individual's condition.** People who helped will naturally want an ongoing update about how the patient is doing. Let them know with a personal website, social-networking page, telephone hotline, or flyer.

❖ **Let people know of any future events.** Tell people about upcoming blood drives and other fundraisers.

Susie's story

After the blood drive, Susie wanted to keep folks updated about David's progress. She contacted a farming machinery company and asked if they had an extra company phone line they'd be willing to contribute for a hotline.

Using this hotline, she could leave a message with updates about David's condition and how people could help. Of course, she always got approval from David and his family.

By calling the hotline, interested friends could check day or night to get news without disturbing David or the family.

11

Note to helpers...
To be sure all of your support is truly kind, take a look at Chapter 6, "Caring without offending" and Chapter 7, "What **to** say, what **not** to say."

Now imagine...

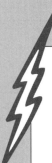

You hear that a blood drive will be held in the company cafeteria for your coworker, Dick. He has been diagnosed with leukemia and will need blood on an ongoing basis.

You've never given blood before, but you and your buddies at work want to do something that will make a difference. You are all a bit nervous, but sign up anyway. As it turns out, giving blood wasn't that hard and you all decide to give again as soon as you can, two months from now.

Or imagine...

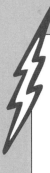

Your neighbor's daughter, Paula, age 16, was in a bad car wreck and received several units of blood. Folks in the neighborhood decide to organize a community blood drive at Paula's school. You want to donate blood, but you learn you're not eligible for several more months because you recently got a tattoo.

Instead, you offer to make and receive phone calls to schedule donors for the drive.

Or imagine this...

A car struck Keith as he was walking to work today. He's now in critical condition, requiring lots of blood. Keith has been the church choir director for years. News of the accident has spread quickly and all of the church members want to help in some way.

Since it's practice night, the distraught choir members gather to prepare for the upcoming service. After many tears and prayers, everyone decides to put together a blood drive for him.

Tom offers to contact the local blood donation center to find out how to coordinate a blood drive right there at the church. Carol will get the word out with flyers, announcements during the church service, a notice on the church website, and a script to be used by callers on the church member phone tree.

Ellen will check with some of the ladies in the church about holding a bake sale as well as serving homemade treats to the blood donors. Mike will work with the men's group to set up the blood drive room, direct parking, and greet folks at the door. Jean and Toby both offer to be available by phone to schedule the donors. Charlie will ask the youth director and the church teens to provide childcare on the day of the drive.

Although the choir members know that Keith's future is out of their hands, they feel better knowing that they can help through this blood drive, the fundraiser, and prayers.

11

CHAPTER TWELVE

Planning a fundraiser or a memorial reception...

In this chapter you'll find answers to...

- How do you plan for a large fundraiser?

- What might you consider when planning a funeral or memorial reception?

- What do you need to do when adding food to a fundraiser?

- What are some menu ideas for fundraising events?

- What are some menu ideas for a funeral or memorial reception?

12

Imagine...

After a terrible car accident, your good friend has huge medical bills. You would like to organize a fundraiser to help cover some of the costs, but you don't know where to start.

Gathering for a big event...

A health crisis or a death brings people together. Sometimes people gather to try to make sense of a tragic event and to show their support by donating blood or raising money for ongoing health-care expenses, a transplant, or scholarships. A reception after a death gives a chance for folks to come together to share their loss and grief and to comfort those left behind. All of these events require lots of volunteers and coordination.

Fundraisers or receptions after a death...

When people feel helpless, a big event gives them a way to contribute. While each community will find its own favorite ways to support each other, here are some examples of common events.

❖ Fundraisers

- Spaghetti dinners
- Pancake dinners
- Dessert buffets
- Comedy shows
- Silent auctions
- Entertainment or talent show
- Fair or carnival

❖ Funeral or memorial receptions

12

Overall planning for a big event...

Regardless of the type of gathering, many of the preparations are the same. However, keep in mind that the feelings that accompany an event will likely be different. A blood drive or a fundraiser brings hope to the future. A reception following a death carries sadness because a life has come to an end.

When planning, consider the following:

❖ **Advertising** For a blood drive or a fundraiser, get the word out (websites, radio or TV announcements, flyers) to ensure good attendance.

> *Funeral or memorial reception:* Media may want to attend if the funeral is for someone well known in the community or if the tragedy has been in the news.

❖ **Budgeting** Of course, the cost of the event and the amount of money available drives the planning. Contact interested organizations (worksites, athletic clubs, neighborhood, service organizations) to gather donated items or financial support.

> *Funeral or memorial reception:* A church or religious organization will often donate the use of the building and a good portion of the reception (cookies, coffee and tea, setup) when a family is a member. Check with the church to find out what portion it will contribute.

❖ **Sponsorship** Businesses, churches, city or county governments, and service organizations can boost the bottom line!

Ask these groups to:

- Donate or give discounts on their services (car washing, gift certificates for raffles, catered meals).

- Buy advertising space (on flyers, posters, or placemats for a fundraising breakfast or dinner).

- Loan equipment (popcorn machine, specialty coffee maker, food steamer, warming table, meat slicer).

- Donate food items (pancake mix, beverages, spaghetti sauce, condiments).

- Donate space (meeting hall, kitchen, parking lot).

❖ **Location** As you plan, estimate the number of people who will be attending. Is the event going to be held outdoors or indoors? Of course, have a back-up plan in case of foul weather.

> ***Funeral or memorial reception:*** Don't assume that all receptions will be held in a church or even indoors. Many are held in a home, a dining hall, or outside at a park.

❖ **Parking** Be sure there are plenty of places to park. If not, have a plan. Find trusted adults to direct traffic and act as valets. If needed, consider asking nearby businesses or homeowners to donate parking spots.

❖ **Time limit** How long will the event last? If it's a pancake breakfast, then it may be only three hours, as opposed to a blood drive that could be an all-day event.

12

❖ **Time of day** When will the event occur? Consider when the most folks would be able to attend.

> *Funeral or memorial reception:* It's becoming more common for funeral services and the accompanying reception to be held in the evening when many working people can attend.

❖ **Theme** Consider giving the event a theme, one that reflects the interests of the person for whom the event is planned. Be sure to get the family's input and permission.

Amber's story

Amber is a nine year old who needs to have a transplant. Her parents have been told that they must come up with a large sum prior to the surgery. The soccer team has decided they will help by putting on a bake sale. Since Amber loves pink, they sell cupcakes, suckers, punch, popcorn balls, and cotton candy—all pink!

> *Funeral or memorial reception:* A reception should reflect the interests, wishes, and the memory of the deceased. It can be as casual as an outdoor picnic or as formal as a fancy buffet.

❖ **Menu** Once the theme and time of day has been chosen, it's relatively easy to plan the menu.

Consider the following:

- Cost, availability, variety, color and balance of food items

- In-season fruits and vegetables

- The temperature of food for food safety

- Quick and easy to serve

- Easy-to-eat foods

- Foods that can be prepared ahead of time

Roberto's story

Roberto, 23, lived and breathed baseball. When he died suddenly, his family decided to have an afternoon outdoor gathering at the park with hot dogs, peanuts, popcorn, cotton candy, lemonade, and his favorite, ice cream!

Friends and family members spent the afternoon both laughing and crying as they remembered Roberto and how much fun he had attending and playing in baseball games.

❖ **Decorations** These can add a lot of fun and flair to any event. Don't forget the tables. Be creative! ***Be sure to get the family's permission.***

> **Funeral or memorial reception:** Typically, flowers will be placed on serving tables and possibly eating tables. Sometimes, the family may request that the decorations revolve around a favorite color or interest of the deceased (pink, green, railroad cars, dinosaurs, sport).

12

Recruiting and coordinating help...

Some large gatherings must be planned within a couple of days, such as immediately following a death. But other times, like with a fundraiser, an event is a month away and folks have more time to plan.

With a big event, you will need a number of leaders and volunteers. If you have lots of help, the big event (spaghetti dinner, car wash, carnival) can then be divided into smaller projects (advertising, decorating, food preparation, donations) with a leader and volunteers for each part.

❖ **Event coordinator** The event coordinator oversees the planning for a big event. She or he will find key contacts (to rally and organize help within various groups) and possibly a project coordinator (to tackle a major job).

❖ **Key contact** Each group that wants to help (neighborhood, school, church, booster club, service organization) will need its own key contact. This person will communicate with the event coordinator, organize the volunteers who wish to help, and keep track of donations.

❖ **Project coordinator** In a big event such as a fundraiser or a reception, someone may step forward and offer to lead a big part (publicity for a blood drive, parking for a large funeral). While this skilled project coordinator may independently do the job, he or she will still be in contact with the event coordinator.

❖ **Volunteers** The volunteers work directly for the key contact within a group or for a project coordinator who is working on a specific job.

Common tasks for a big event...

Regardless of the size of your event, many tasks will need to be considered.

Deciding what needs to be done...

❖ Talk with the individual or family about how people can help.

❖ Make a master list of possible projects (blood drive, pet care, transportation, funeral reception).

❖ Decide what work volunteers will do and what jobs should be hired out with donated funds (catered food, housecleaning, remodeling to make the home wheelchair-accessible).

❖ Break down big projects into smaller parts.

❖ Don't forget to plan for breakdown and cleanup after the event.

❖ Make up a master calendar to organize efforts.

❖ Publicize the event.

Gathering the folks to help...

❖ Make a list of the groups or organizations that might be interested in helping.

❖ Notify the groups regarding the crisis.

❖ Find a leader within each group to coordinate all volunteers and work.

12

❖   Communicate the list of jobs that the family needs.

❖   Ask each group what they want to do to help.

❖   Find out how frequently each group can help.

❖   Make a list of volunteers who have offered to help. Include names, home and e-mail addresses, and home and cell phone numbers.

❖   Find the right job at the right time for the right person.

Scheduling the folks to help...

❖   Figure out the number of people needed to help with each job.

❖   For jobs requiring shifts, determine the needed time periods (8 A.M. to 11 A.M.) and the number of people needed for each shift.

❖   Contact and schedule folks to help. Be sure volunteers know exactly when and where to show up.

Tracking donations...

❖   Set up a bank account for money donations.

❖   Collect money donations for needed items (food, house cleaning, remodeling supplies).

❖   Coordinate donated flight miles.

❖   Keep the books.

Communicate, communicate, communicate!

❖ Keep communication going between all leaders, volunteers, and all efforts.

❖ Assign someone to be the contact person when people have questions and problems. Be sure all volunteers have this person's number.

❖ Make calls to remind volunteers to show up.

❖ Give maps, directions, and essential information to volunteers.

❖ Ask volunteers to report back when they have completed a job (taken a meal, given a ride, shoveled the walk, built a ramp).

❖ Ask volunteers to report if they have any concerns (notice a problem, see something else that the family needs).

❖ Troubleshoot when there are problems.

❖ Stir up enthusiasm for the project.

❖ Thank volunteers with either a written note or a small remembrance of the event (homemade magnet, Christmas ornament, personalized candy) for making a difference!

Just add food — the essential ingredient to any event...

People will always hover around a table of food! A simple pancake breakfast, a spaghetti dinner, or a potluck will bring people from miles away. Folks count on the aroma, the flavors, and the sounds of people chatting. Food brings a bit of festivity, a sense of community, and a chance for people to

12

reach out to others for something good. Of course, after a death, people will gather to pay their respects. In all of these situations, food is central as a comfort measure and sometimes as a necessity when folks have come from far away.

Handling all of the food details for a big event...

When a large group of people needs to be fed, it takes lots of planning, coordination, and helpers. In this case, you cannot have too much help. If you can, find someone who has had experience coordinating food for a large event.

Putting together a plan first!

If you are counting on a bunch of people eating, thorough planning will make all the difference.

❖   **Decide if the event should be catered or home-cooked.** This decision will depend on whether or not an organization has offered to sponsor the event, if enough money has been donated, or if volunteers are willing or able to cook.

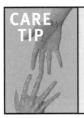

CARE TIP

If you decide your group will do the cooking, be sure to find a kitchen that has been officially inspected and approved for cooking for large groups (church, fire station, school).

❖ **If catering the event, contract with the restaurant or the catering company.** Sometimes having an event professionally catered is the best option because of limited help or lack of experience. Catering services can include food preparation, setup, serving and cleanup, or just the food preparation, delivery, and pickup after the event.

❖ **Come up with a menu.** Once you develop the overall plan for the event, choosing the menu is easy. Of course, the food items will vary depending on the event (fundraiser or funeral reception, casual or formal). See "Feeding the body and soul," page 165.

❖ **Decide if food will be prepared in a large central kitchen or in homes.** Sometimes if space is limited, it's best to give people a recipe and ask them to prepare the dish at home. Or, if a huge kitchen is available, the group may decide to have folks prepare food there. This may be best, especially if extreme cleanliness or a special diet is needed (for immune deficiency due to chemotherapy, for severe allergies to peanuts).

❖ **Make a timeline.** A timeline helps ensure that everything is ready at the right time. Remember to include tasks that are important even before anything is cooked (emptying and cleaning refrigerators and freezers, shopping for foods, cleaning the fruits and vegetables).

❖ **Find leaders to be in charge of all of the food-related jobs.** For a very large event, you may need many leaders for each big job (shopping for the food, food preparation, setting the tables, decorating the room, serving, cleaning up).

❖ **Plan ahead for the breakdown and cleanup of the event.** Arrange for a fresh crew of volunteers who are coming just for the cleanup because this is often the hardest part!

12

Getting things ready before the food arrives...

Be ready for the food when it comes! This is easier said than done. If you can, find someone who has had experience coordinating food for a large event.

❖ **Calculate quantities of ingredients and supplies.** This is not an easy task. Be sure to get help from someone experienced in preparing food for large groups. How much people will eat and drink depends on many factors (weather, males or females, age, location). Don't forget the condiments (salt, pepper, sugar, mustard, mayonnaise, ketchup).

❖ **Make two separate shopping lists.** First, make a list of non-perishable items that can be purchased ahead of time. Second, make a list of those items that are perishable (fruit, vegetables, milk) and need to be bought at the last minute so they are fresh.

❖ **Collect money donations for food items.** Sometimes it's easier and safer for folks (who are not skilled in cooking) to just donate money to buy what is needed. Designate someone to keep the detailed records of all donations as well as expenses.

❖ **Prepare a detailed work order.** What should you prepare first, second, or at the last minute, for example?

❖ **Shop for groceries and supplies.** If the event is large, more than one person and one vehicle may be needed. Bring someone along who is strong!

❖ **Find back-up refrigerators.** Since large quantities of food will be coming, one refrigerator will not be enough. Find other refrigerators close by, if possible.

❖ **Clean out refrigerators.** Spotless refrigerators will help keep the food clean and safe for your guests.

❖ **Find back-up freezers.** Once again, with large quantities of food, one freezer may not be enough. Check with the church, service organizations, corporations, or neighbors and friends to see if they have extra freezer space. People may want to bake or cook food ahead of time as their schedule allows. Also, many events will require ice or ice rings for punch. If additional freezers are not possible, consider large ice chests. Remember, these will only keep foods cold for a short time.

❖ **Clean out freezers and ice chests.** Again, only put food and ice in a clean freezer or ice chest.

❖ **Anticipate food cooking, baking, and rewarming.** If a full meal is planned, you will likely need several stovetops and ovens. Though churches may have more than one, consider lining up several neighbors' ovens if you are hosting a reception in a home. Or, you could have warming trays, chafing dishes, and portable roasting ovens available.

As you plan your menu, limit the numbers of food items that require last-minute heating. Regardless of how much planning you do, some people will still come with a homemade dish to warm up at the last minute.

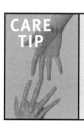

CARE TIP

Even churches may have limited food storage and cooking space if multiple events are occurring around the same time. Be sure to check with the church office regarding the schedule for the kitchen.

12

❖ **Plan for additional storage space.** When a reception will be held in a home, storage is always an issue. Consider using a garage that has been emptied. Set up folding tables or picnic tables, or make them from doors or wooden planks on top of saw horses. Tarps laid on the ground may provide short-term clean and dry storage space for unopened packages and beverage containers.

❖ **Gather equipment.** Food preparation often requires a variety of equipment (trays, serving utensils, warming trays, chafing dishes, portable roasting ovens, meat slicers, peelers, knives, electric knives, mixers, bowls, measuring cups and spoons, pitchers). Check to be sure the facility or home has what you need. If you need to borrow equipment, be sure each piece is labeled.

❖ **Anticipate the need for electrical outlets.** If electrical warmers and coffee makers will be used, find all outlets. Try them out first so you don't blow fuses in the middle of the event.

❖ **Clear off counter space.** Volunteers will need plenty of room to prepare food. Check to be sure the counters are not stacked up with unnecessary items. If so, find out where you can temporarily store the items until your event is over.

❖ **Find someone who is ready and able to answer questions.** This person should be experienced with food preparation and cooking as well as packaging and delivering foods. This is a great job for someone who might not be able to make and deliver meals (due to poor mobility, a disability, family situation), but would like to offer advice over the phone.

❖ **Keep a list of people who bring food donations.** Though family members should not feel the need to send a note in response, this list may bring some comfort in the future.

❖ **Plan for the distribution or donation of leftovers.** Check with the family to see if they will want part or all of the leftover food. If they don't, make arrangements ahead of time with a nearby shelter or youth center. Each organization may have special requirements for the food they can accept.

Large Gathering Supply List

Disposable items

- ☐ Disposable table covers (These plastic or paper table covers make cleanup easy.)
- ☐ Disposable serving bowls or trays
- ☐ Paper goods (facial tissue, toilet paper, napkins, paper towels)
- ☐ Disposable plates, cups, bowls
- ☐ Plasticware (forks, spoons, knives)
- ☐ Storage bags or containers (Great for leftovers!)
- ☐ Plastic wrap and aluminum foil (Essential for packaging up leftovers.)
- ☐ Ice or re-freezable blue ice (for beverages or keeping perishables cold)
- ☐ Trash bags (small and large)
- ☐ Dishwashing detergent
- ☐ Disposable wipes

Reusable items

- ☐ Tablecloths (Many churches have tablecloths they use for special occasions. Also, some families may want to use a tablecloth that has some special memory.)

continued on next page

12

Large Gathering Supply List (continued)

- ☐ Serving bowls, platters, trays
- ☐ Serving pieces (large spoons, large serving forks, cake or pie servers, spatulas, knives)
- ☐ Punch bowl & ladle
- ☐ Salt & pepper shakers/grinders
- ☐ Baskets
- ☐ Condiment dishes
- ☐ Candles
- ☐ Table center pieces, flower arrangements
- ☐ Serving carts (These can either be fancy or a cafeteria-type cart that can be used for moving food from a kitchen to the reception area.)
- ☐ Individual trays or tray-like plates (These are ideal when there is limited seating space.)
- ☐ Silverware/flatware (Most churches have forks, spoons, and knives that can go through the dishwasher.)
- ☐ China service (Many churches and families have place settings of plates, cups, and bowls that they will want to use.)
- ☐ Dishcloths
- ☐ Tarps (These may come in handy to put down if food is being stored on a garage floor or on large picnic tables.)

Miscellaneous food items

- ☐ Condiments (Don't forget the salt, pepper, sugar, mustard, mayonnaise, ketchup, syrup, soy sauce, hot sauce, or barbeque sauce.)

Preparing and assembling the food...

If you are "doing it yourself" instead of using costly catering, you will have lots to do.

❖ **Cut and slice foods and assemble trays (meat, cheese, veggie, fruit, cookie trays).** Preparing takes a lot more time than you might imagine.

❖ **Make salads, sandwich fillings, sandwiches, casseroles, vegetables, desserts, or breads.** The more items that are washed, cut, and mixed ahead of time, the smoother the assembly will go.

❖ **Prepare punch, coffee, or other beverages.** The weather that day will impact the amount and type of beverage needed. On a cold day, get the coffee going early. On a hot day, have plenty of cold drinks and ice set up.

❖ **Collect any food that volunteers may have prepared at home.** For some people, it will be easier and more practical to prepare food (roasts, cookies, casseroles, sandwich fillings, salads) at home and bring it to the site for further assembly. It's helpful to have someone ready and waiting who will label and add instructions for reheating or last minute preparation.

❖ **Deliver food to the event.** Remind people who are bringing hot or liquid items to protect their car. Avoid spills by securing containers, placing them in boxes, or laying down plastic tarps to cover the seats, floor, or trunk. This will prevent any last-minute chaos with folks needing help cleaning up messes.

12

❖ **Fill trays, serving dishes, or pitchers.** Food that was prepared in large quantities will likely need to be divided onto trays or into serving dishes. Be sure to have people ready to do this.

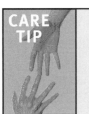

CARE TIP Stress the necessity for thorough cleanliness and safe food storage. This may include reminders to helpers not to prepare food if they are ill, to wash hands frequently, and to keep foods either at cold temperatures or at hot temperatures to ensure safe storage. ***This is an important point!*** Families in crisis cannot afford the added stress of an illness transmitted by food.

Setting up the room...

❖ **Arrange the buffet tables for easy flow.** Be sure that there is room for folks to go down both sides of the table to speed things up.

❖ **Spread out the food tables.** To avoid crowding, consider placing the food in different parts of the room, yard, park, etc. Folks will always gravitate to the food tables.

❖ **Consider the ease of serving or proximity to kitchen.** Set out the hottest and sloppiest foods closer to the kitchen.

❖ **Set up the event site.** Some events, like fundraisers, might have a theme to decorate around. Other events, like a memorial service, might not. Bottom line, make the event site warm and welcoming.

❖ **Set tables for reception.** This can include putting on tablecloths, plates, cups, napkins, silverware, flowers, tea or coffee service, sugar and creamer, or serving utensils.

❖ **Set up a children's eating area.** Sometimes families will lay out clean blankets or newspapers on the floor to make cleanup easy and keep damage from spills to a minimum.

Shellisa's story

Six-year-old Shellisa died after a severe asthma attack. The gathering after her funeral was supposed to be held outside in a friend's backyard. Unfortunately, it rained all afternoon, chasing the folks who came to the reception into the house. While the adults gathered upstairs, the many children played downstairs.

There were not enough chairs to go around, so when it was time to eat, blankets were spread out on the floor to make a comfortable eating place for the kids.

Serving the food...

Anticipate that some serving jobs require lots of lifting, pushing, coordination, and energy, while others can be done with little movement. Be sure to match the right people with the right serving job.

❖ **Serve food or tend buffet table.** Someone needs to constantly be watching to see when food and trays need to be refilled. For big events, a crew should be ready to jump into action when notified.

❖ **Deliver food and beverages to food or buffet tables.** Safety is important. Find plenty of sturdy carts to wheel the food to the tables.

12

❖ **Pour coffee, tea, punch, or other beverages.** This is the perfect job for someone who needs "light duty." Refilling the heavy beverage coffee pots or punch bowls, however, should go to someone else.

❖ **Serve food and beverages to the family members or to anyone too feeble to stand in line.** Often family members are too occupied to think of themselves or to break away from conversation to get something to eat or drink. Have someone watching and ready to attend to family members or to those who need extra assistance.

Cleaning up after the event...

While cleanup is not the most glamorous job, it is essential. Typically, the volunteers who have been there for the event are now fatigued and it is important to bring on fresh volunteers to clean up. Unfortunately, this is the one job that is often forgotten.

❖ **Bring dirty dishes, silverware, and trays back to the kitchen.** Cleanup should begin as soon as the event starts. Don't let things pile up.

❖ **Wash dishes, trays, silverware, glassware, etc.** If a commercial dishwasher (in a church or service organization) is being used, be sure someone is trained ahead of time to operate the equipment and to follow safe washing practices.

❖ **Clean tablecloths.** If the cloths are plastic and will be reused, wipe them down, dry, and fold them. If they are cloth, plan to spot-treat, wash, iron, and fold them. Or, send the tablecloths to a dry cleaner.

❖ **Break down tables and stack chairs.** Some facilities will have their own directions for how the room/area should be left.

❖ **Get rid of trash.** This includes not only gathering it up, but also taking it out to dumpsters. Be sure to have plenty of plastic bags and volunteers ready to make this job easier.

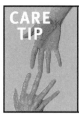

CARE TIP

Be sure to have volunteers assigned to collect and remove trash right from the beginning of the event! This will not only make the final cleanup easier, but it will also make the entire event run smoothly.

❖ **Re-wrap and package leftover foods.** Have plenty of foil, plastic wrap, re-closable plastic bags, and disposable containers available to make cleanup and distribution of leftovers easy.

❖ **Distribute remaining food.** Leftovers can either be a curse or a blessing for the distressed individual or family. If leftovers are packaged in smaller portions, family members won't have to worry about mealtime later on. However, check to be sure the family wants them and also that they have enough freezer or storage space available. If not, find someone living close by who does.

If the family does not want some or all of the food, deliver leftovers to places where it can be used (shelters, youth centers, food distribution centers, employee lounge at a family member's worksite).

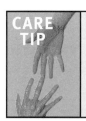

CARE TIP

Disposable containers make cleanup easy and keep the family from having to return serving dishes.

12

Menu ideas for fundraising events...

A fundraiser becomes "a recipe for success" when food is added to the mix. The local favorite fare (ham and bean supper, burritos, clam bake, Chinese chop suey, sloppy joes) will draw people from across the city or from miles away. Consider combining fundraisers (car wash and bake sale, blood drive and barbeque, spaghetti dinner and raffle, craft sale and homemade soup-and-salad buffet) for different appetites and an even bigger crowd.

Don't give up if you don't like to cook. You can pull in businesses that will do the work for you. For example, a pizza restaurant might be willing to donate a portion of their profits on a given night. Then, instead of cooking, you just need to widely advertise to get folks in the door. Or, you might find a restaurant that would be willing to donate, discount, or even cater as part of a fundraising event. Check online for more fundraising ideas and helpful suggestions.

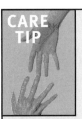

CARE TIP Surprisingly, most food fundraisers are much more profitable when you ask for donations rather than a set price. For example, instead of charging $6.00 for a spaghetti dinner, just ask for a donation. While some folks may not put in enough to cover costs, others, with the meaningful purpose in mind, will be more than generous.

Blood drive...

Blood donors need refreshments and nutrition immediately after giving blood. Blood collection centers typically provide juice and store-bought cookies for donors. However, if the blood drive is held at a worksite, church, or community center, this is a great opportunity to add on a fundraiser (home-baked goods, all-day pancake feasts, barbeques, ice cream sundaes).

Spaghetti or local favorite dinner...

Choose a menu that can be easily prepared for large groups (fish fries, barbeques, fish boils, ethnic foods). Sometimes, a local restaurant will provide the food and the fixings as a full donation or at a reduced price in exchange for the advertising.

Dessert buffet following entertainment...

Add a dessert to a fun event (talent show, musical, play, poetry or story recital, concert). No talent? Don't worry. Silly skits, spoofs, or comedy "roasts" can be hilarious!

Bake sale...

Everyone loves a homemade treat! With the family's approval, consider organizing a bake sale. A bake sale is a great addition to any other fund-raising event.

❖ **Cookies** Sell one at a time or package them up to sell in small or larger quantities.

❖ **Brownies** Yum!

❖ **Candies** Homemade is always the best!

❖ **Popcorn** Caramel, flavored, plain, in balls

❖ **Homemade cookie or cake mixes in a jar** Advertise these as the perfect gift to have on hand to give for birthdays, "pick-me-ups," or teacher gifts.

12

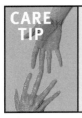

CARE TIP Mixes in a jar are a perfect project for kids to put together. Be sure to have adult supervision and to insist on thorough hand washing.

❖ **Homemade dry soup mixes in a jar** Try bean, noodle, or potato. Check online for recipes.

❖ **Homemade beverage mixes in a jar** Flavored coffee, spiced tea, or mulled-wine mixes are good choices.

❖ **Cakes** Sell whole or by the slice.

❖ **Pies** Who doesn't love a piece of homemade pie?

❖ **Breads** These can be yeast breads (whole wheat, cheese, Italian) or sweet (banana, pumpkin, zucchini).

❖ **Jams and jellies** Decorate the jar with a bright ribbon.

❖ **Salsas and sauces** Heat to a safe temperature and seal properly.

❖ **Pizza** Serve it hot and by the slice, or sell it ready to toss in the oven.

❖ **Pre-cooked specialty items** Consider homemade meatballs, soups, barbequed meats or local favorites.

❖ **Ice cream sundaes** Perfect on a hot day.

❖ **Hot chocolate** Delightful on a cold and snowy day.

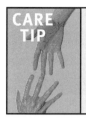

CARE TIP

Don't forget extra paper plates, napkins, plastic wrap, aluminum foil, tape or labels, and marking pens.

Pancake breakfast or supper...

The old-fashioned pancake breakfast is one of the easiest to put together. The ingredients are inexpensive and simple, so making a profit is assured if you get the people in the door. Plus, this event is a time where folks who haven't seen each other in a while can gather for a good cause.

❖ **Pancake mix** The just-add-water kind is easiest and works great!

❖ **Seasonings** A touch of cinnamon is a delicious addition!

❖ **Pancake griddles** Some large service organizations or churches often have these built in or they can be rented.

❖ **Batter dispenser** This is a handy device that makes uniform-shaped pancakes and speeds up the process!

❖ **Sausage or bacon** You can now find these precooked and then you just warm them up.

❖ **Fruit** Fresh colorful fruit, when in season, is a great option.

❖ **Juices** Orange juice is traditional, but others are certainly fine.

12

- ❖ **Syrup** As well as maple, have blueberry, strawberry, apricot, and low-sugar syrups on hand.

- ❖ **Butter** Butter/margarine can come in single-serving packages or you can just put sticks or tubs on the table.

- ❖ **Additional beverages** Milk, coffee, tea

- ❖ **Cream and cream substitutes**

- ❖ **Sugar and sugar substitutes**

- ❖ **Tablecloths** Large rolls of colored paper or plastic make for an easy cleanup.

- ❖ **Napkins**

- ❖ **Plates and cups**

- ❖ **Flatware or plasticware** Forks, knives, spoons

Keith's story

Keith, a beloved elementary school teacher, has recently been diagnosed with a severe case of multiple sclerosis. Since his vision has been affected, he is not able to teach and has been forced to go on disability. His family is suddenly in danger of losing their home.

Keith's fellow teachers want to do something to help. As a fundraiser, they decide to put on a comical variety show for the community. Each family is asked to bring a dessert to share as well as cash to donate for Keith's expenses. The event is a rip-roaring success and the proceeds help meet the mortgage payments for a couple of months!

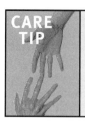

CARE TIP

Whether you're holding a garage sale, car wash, carnival, or other fundraiser, the workers will likely need food and drinks to keep them going. Don't forget to feed them!

Food for a funeral or memorial reception...

A memorial or funeral reception is an important part of saying goodbye. People who gather may have come from far away. So, a comforting reception brings support to the family and friends at a very difficult time. Helping with the reception provides an opportunity for people to help when they really can't do much to take away someone's pain.

When you plan the reception, consider the time of day, the location of the service, and the numbers expected to attend. While many receptions are held in a church after a religious service, others are held in a funeral home, reception hall, or a private home. Some families may choose to keep the reception casual and hold the remembrance in a park or a private backyard.

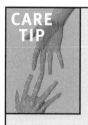

CARE TIP

Don't duplicate efforts. If the deceased had a religious membership, first check with the church or synagogue to see if members are planning to provide a reception following the service. If they are, then perhaps friends can help supplement with additional food dishes.

A reception following a service can be as simple as a tray of cookies or as complex as a full buffet. Depending on the time of day and if folks have come from far away, a hardier menu may be needed.

12

❖ **Prepared sandwiches** Pre-made, easy-to-eat sandwiches are perfect for a very large gathering. They will prevent the long lines that occur when people are forced to assemble their own.

❖ **Meat and cheese trays** These are great for building your own sandwiches if you have small groups. Be sure to have rolls or bread cut and ready to go.

❖ **Condiments** Don't forget to include mustard and ketchup, mayonnaise, butter or margarine, salt & pepper, or whatever special condiments (soy sauce, hot sauce, barbeque sauce) are needed for your menu.

❖ **Relish trays** Include raw vegetables, pickles, peppers, and olives, etc.

❖ **Main dish casseroles** These will vary depending on the family and community's tastes.

❖ **Meat or fish dishes** Again, this is a family preference, but common choices might be ham, chicken, beef or pork roasts, and fish dishes.

❖ **Traditional favorites** Of course, each family and community has its own traditional foods that add special comfort.

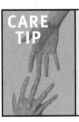

CARE TIP

Sometimes, the family might request to have a special recipe that the deceased person loved. If not, check to see if they would like any special foods included.

❖ **Vegetable dishes** Everyone appreciates these and vegetarians will doubly appreciate you.

❖ **Fruit trays** Whatever is in season will work!

❖ **Salads** Consider tossed, potato, three-bean, seafood, pasta salads, or coleslaw.

❖ **Desserts** Cakes, pies, brownies, bars, cookies, etc., can top off a meal or be served alone.

❖ **Drinks** Have plenty of punch, iced tea, coffee, tea, soda, lemonade, juices, or bottled water available.

❖ **Ice** A must for both drinks and food storage! For outdoor events, be sure you have plenty to keep perishable foods cold.

❖ **Sugar and cream for coffee or tea** Don't forget the substitutes for sugar and cream (non-fat, flavored).

Note to helpers...
To be sure all of your support is truly kind,
take a look at Chapter 6, "Caring without offending"
and Chapter 7, "What *to* say, what *not* to say."

12

Now imagine...

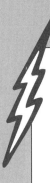

You want to help with the upcoming spaghetti dinner fundraiser, but because of your bad knees, you have trouble doing a lot of walking. You offer to make the table centerpieces at home. You ask a friend to pick up the supplies you will need so you can get started working. After you've put the centerpieces together, you ask another friend to deliver them to the event hall.

On the night of the fundraiser, you arrive to see the hall filled with happy folks enjoying the spaghetti dinner. It's fun to see that your contribution has added a bit of fun to the celebration.

Or imagine...

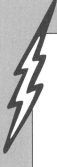

Sadly, Paul, a beloved science teacher in the local elementary school, has suddenly died. You have been close friends for years with Paul and his wife, Susan. You know that he is a member of a local church, so you contact them to see if they need help with the funeral reception.

The church is prepared to provide a reception with homemade cookies and beverages. The women's group from the church plans to help with all of the serving. You know that many folks from the neighborhood and school will be attending and will want to contribute in some way. You ask if it would be okay for these groups to provide veggie, fruit, and sandwich trays, and the church agrees.

You decide that it will be easiest to just collect donations to buy the food trays from the local deli. Everyone is thrilled to help. The money you collect not only covers the cost of the trays, but also is enough for a number of fun science books to be given in Paul's name for the school library.

Or imagine this...

Jennie, a 14-year-old member of the local horseback-riding club, suddenly started having seizures. Unfortunately, the doctors found that a brain tumor was the cause. Jennie immediately had surgery, but now has balance problems. As a result, she will have a long recovery and will need lots of therapy. Her club wants to put on a dessert buffet fundraiser that includes a horseshow performance.

12

Her friends put out the word by e-mail and through flyers posted at the church, school, and local businesses. They find a local restaurant that is willing to donate some of its prized cheesecakes and a favorite coffee shop that will donate the coffee.

The club members plan the performance and spend lots of time practicing to make the event great. The parents volunteer to serve and clean up so that the kids can concentrate on getting their horses groomed and ready.

When the big day comes, Jennie and her parents are able to attend and enjoy the show. The event is very successful, raising several thousand dollars for Jennie's therapy costs.

Thoughts to leave you with...

Dear Friends,

We all know that crises will strike. It's just part of life. When we find our friends or family dazed and alone, we've each been given a unique opportunity to become an "everyday hero." While we may struggle to do or say the right thing, we need to remember that it is the thought and kindness behind our words and deeds that really matter.

We know that you "everyday heroes" are out there! We would love to hear your success stories. You can find us at www.WhenCrisisStrikes.com.

Warmly,
Allidah and Bonnie

PART V
Additional resources...

Forms to help when...

In this section you'll find useful forms...

- Letting people know...

- People willing to help...

- Food preparation and delivery...

- Blood drive schedule...

Letting people know...

Who was involved? (name/s)	
What happened? (accident, serious illness, death)	
Condition? (alive, hurt, conscious, unconscious, talking)	
When was it? (day, time)	
Where did it happen? (in town, out of town, work, school)	
Where are they now? (name of hospital, home)	
Should people call? (yes, no, check with nurses' station first)	
Where can people call or log on to get more information? (hospital unit & number, contact name & number, hotline number, website address)	
Where/when can people leave messages? (phone, e-mail, website, social-networking site)	
Should people visit? (yes, no, check with nurses' station first)	
When is it a good time to visit? (not at all, morning, afternoon, evening)	
How can people help? (baking, cooking, visiting, transportation, caring for kids, pets, home, yard, donations)	

A

People willing to help...

Name	Phone #s	Relationship (neighbor, relative, work, church)	Type of help (meals, childcare, pet care, transportation, yard, house cleaning, fixing ramps for wheelchair)	Day/Dates	Time/s available (mornings, afternoons, evenings)

B

Food preparation and delivery...

Total # of people to be served: _____

Family member names	Infant	Toddler	Preschool	School age	Adolescent	Adult	Older adult

Additional guests to be served: _____   # Children: _____   # Adults: _____

What: ☐ Breakfast   ☐ Lunch   ☐ Dinner   ☐ Other/Snack

Food allergies to consider: _____

Food likes and dislikes: _____

C

Disposable plates: ☐ Yes ☐ No Disposable cups: ☐ Yes ☐ No Napkins: ☐ Yes ☐ No

Plasticware: ☐ Yes ☐ No Serving utensils: ☐ Yes ☐ No

Help set up: ☐ Yes ☐ No Help clean up: ☐ Yes ☐ No Bring back empty serving dishes/utensils: ☐ Yes ☐ No

When: Day: _____ Date: _____ Time: _____ Meal time: _____ ☐ AM ☐ PM

Best time to deliver: _____ Call before delivery? ☐ Yes ☐ No Phone # to call: _____

Name of family contact at hospital: _____ Other instructions: _____

Where to deliver: ☐ Hospital ☐ Home ☐ Other location: _____

Hospital: _____

Travel & parking directions: _____

_____

Home address: _____

Travel & parking directions: _____

_____

Other location: _____

Travel & parking directions: _____

_____

Have questions? Call: _____ at (phone #) _____

Blood drive schedule...

Start time & donor chair #	Name	Phone #'s (home, work, cell)	Address	Relation to patient (relative, neighbor, school, work)	Donor info (blood type, previous/ frequent donor, bone marrow testing)	Possible bone marrow donor?	Misc. (sick, taking meds, referred to center for ?s)
(Time) #1							
#2							
#3							
(Time) #1							
#2							
#3							

D

Index

Please share your story!

Hey, you "Everyday Hero!" We would love to hear from you! Tell us what you said or did that made a difference for someone going through a bad time.

Or, has there been an "Everyday Hero" in your life? Tell us what they said or did that put a smile on your face or brought you a bit of comfort.

Your ideas or story might be just the answer for someone else. Please keep your story to 2000 characters (online) or to one typed page.

Contact us online: Go to *www.WhenCrisisStrikes.com*

Contact us by mail: Good Neighbors Publishing LLC
24325 Winder Place
Golden, CO 80403

We need your permission to use your idea!

We will assume that if you send us your story and check the 1st box below, you are giving us permission to use your idea either on our website, in a talk or future book, or for our book promotion. We will *not* use any part of your name unless you check the 2nd box below.

☐ **Check here if you have read and agree to the permission statement.**

☐ **Check here if we can use your first name with your idea or story.**

Please print clearly!

Name: _____

Address: _____

City: _____ State: _____ ZIP Code: _____

Country: _____

Order Form

Order online: *www.WhenCrisisStrikes.com*

Order by mail: Complete and mail the order form below. Include your personal check or money order, payable to Good Neighbors Publishing LLC. Send payment to:

Good Neighbors Publishing LLC
24325 Winder Place
Golden, Colorado 80403

Yes! Send me: Quantity _____ **@ $27.95 each.**   Subtotal: $ _____
(*For quantities of 5 or more, please see website for rates.*)
Add Postage and Handling **@ $7.50.**   Subtotal: $ _____
Add **$1.50** for each additional book   Subtotal: $ _____
Colorado residents add **$1.40 per book** (5%) for state taxes.
                                                  Subtotal: $ _____
                                        Total enclosed: $ _____

Please do not send cash. Sorry, no C.O.D.s. Please allow 2 weeks for delivery.
Payment by: Check: _____
              Money Order: _____
              Credit Card: _____ Card Type: _____
Credit Card #: _____ Expiration Date: _____ Security ID #: _____
                                                  (3 digit # on back of card)

Please print:
Name: _____ Organization: _____

Address: _____

City: _____ State: _____ ZIP code: _____

Daytime phone (for order questions): _____

Ship to (if different from above):
Name: _____ Organization: _____

Address: _____

City: _____ State: _____ ZIP code: _____

When Crisis Strikes... is a perfect gift for anyone who wants to help.